Oxford Chemistry Series

General Editors
P. W. ATKINS   J. S. E. HOLKER   A. K. HOLLIDAY

D1480358

Oxford Chemistry Series

J. STAUNTON

UNIVERSITY LECTURER IN CHEMISTRY AND
FELLOW OF ST. JOHN'S COLLEGE, CAMBRIDGE

Primary metabolism:

a mechanistic approach

1978

Clarendon Press · Oxford

Oxford University Press, Walton Street, Oxford OX2 6DP

OXFORD LONDON GLASGOW NEW YORK
TORONTO MELBOURNE WELLINGTON CAPE TOWN
IBADAN NAIROBI DAR ES SALAAM LUSAKA
KUALA LUMPUR SINGAPORE JAKARTA HONG KONG TOKYO
DELHI BOMBAY CALCUTTA MADRAS KARACHI

© OXFORD UNIVERSITY PRESS 1978

British Library Cataloguing in Publication Data

Staunton, J
    Primary metabolism.–(Oxford chemistry series).
    1. Metabolism
    I. Title II. Series
    574.1′33   QH521   77–30367

ISBN 0–19–855460–5

Typeset in Northern Ireland by Universities Press, Belfast.
Printed in Great Britain by R. Clay & Co. Ltd., Bungay, Suffolk

Editor's foreword

TRADITIONALLY the chemistry of essential life processes (primary metabolism) has been the province of the biochemist while the study of non-essential, species-specific metabolites (secondary metabolism) has provided a fertile field of study for the organic chemist. However, we now know that primary and secondary metabolism are closely inter-related and that a knowledge of both is essential to give a balanced picture of this important area of chemistry. Despite this, undergraduate courses in natural-product chemistry frequently ignore the fundamental life processes which provide the starting materials for the biosynthesis of the more exotic secondary metabolites.

Dr. Staunton is an organic chemist who has made many original contributions to the field of secondary metabolism. In this book he presents the field of primary metabolism in terms of the concepts which are familiar to the organic chemist and which enable him to correlate enzyme-mediated reactions with his knowledge of *in vitro* chemistry. He thus sees that chemical reactions in the living system are controlled by the same fundamental disciplines as other chemical reactions. This treatment is not only reassuring to the organic chemist but it generates new ideas in both biological chemistry and synthetic chemistry based on biological analogies (biomimetic synthesis). The field is thus extremely challenging.

This book together with the companion books in the Oxford Chemistry Series, *Metals and metabolism* (OCS 26) by D. A. Phipps and *Secondary metabolism* (OCS 27) by J. Mann provide the broad coverage of biological chemistry which should find a place in any modern undergraduate course.

J. S. E. H.

Preface

Man has used natural chemical processes, for example, in the two basic industries of brewing and breadmaking, since before recorded history, and so it was inevitable that from its inception one of the main interests of the modern science of chemistry should be the chemical processes of life. Progress was slow until the early nineteenth century when, as a result of improved techniques of purification, natural products were isolated at an ever increasing rate. Since that time an enormous effort has been directed towards the elucidation of the structure and the synthesis of these compounds. The early development of the subject (which we now know as organic chemistry) was largely determined by work in this field. Thus on the practical side the challenge of tackling compounds and mixtures of increasing complexity provided a powerful impetus to the search for improved practical techniques. Even more important, however, was the stimulating effect of natural product research on the development of the theoretical side of the subject. As compounds of established structure increased in number and diversity, patterns of reactivity emerged which could not be adequately explained by existing theory. Modern ideas of conformational analysis and non-benzenoid aromaticity, for example, were sparked off in this way.

Organic chemists were interested not only in the structures of natural products but also in the reactions which lead to their formation *in vivo*—witness the many biosynthetic speculations which can be found in the chemical literature going back to the early years of this century. However, they neglected to follow up this interest by doing experiments, and the foundations of experimental work on the reactions of living systems were laid by a new breed of chemist, the biochemist. As a consequence an unfortunate dichotomy developed in which two closely related branches of chemistry followed parallel courses but with regretably little cross-fertilization.

This state of affairs continued until the middle of this century when the course of natural product research was profoundly altered by two developments which had their origins outside the subject. First spectroscopic machines were refined by physicists to the stage where they could be applied routinely to the study of organic molecules. As a result the classical methods of solving natural product structures were superceded, and with them went much of the challenge of this line of research. The second major development was the increased availability of isotopes, particularly carbon and tritium. With these the organic chemist could conveniently seek answers to long-standing questions concerning the biosynthesis of natural products by carrying out incorporation experiments with living systems. Many grasped this opportunity. Having tested the water and found it to their liking they have waded deeper and deeper into the biochemical sea and nowadays it is common to find organic chemists studying biological reactions employing in the process the latest and most sophisticated techniques of practical biochemistry.

This book has been written as an introduction to this area of overlap between organic chemistry and biochemistry which has grown in recent years. It deals with the pathways of primary metabolism, that is, those which are fundamental to life in that they provide the materials and energy used by living cells for their maintenance and growth. Though attention is focused on the chemical aspects of the reactions it is hoped that the treatment will interest biochemists as well as organic chemists.

In the early chapters selected key processes are treated in isolation with emphasis on their mechanism and energetics. In later chapters the biochemical perspective is emphasized to show how the individual reactions mesh together to form a metabolic pathway.

As the title indicates, a mechanistic approach is adopted in the treatment of reactions. Since mechanism is interpreted in different ways in the various branches of chemistry, it seems wise to explain here in what sense the word is used in this book: we shall consider what intermediates are or might be involved in each process and also the nature of the electronic shifts which take place when one intermediate is converted to another. This approach has been used with great success to systematize the diverse reactions of organic chemistry and has brought considerable benefits to the teaching of that subject. In the present context it will be used to show how many apparently unrelated chemical processes are in fact closely related in mechanism; to emphasize the relationship between biochemical processes and analogous chemical reactions; to show that by considering the mechanism of biological reactions organic chemists can design novel chemical processes which are of use in synthetic organic chemistry.

One aspect of mechanism which will not be treated in depth is the question of reaction kinetics. In other words we shall not consider in detail which stage of a multistage reaction is rate determining or how the individual steps might be catalysed by the enzyme. These considerations are of course essential to a complete understanding of the mechanism of any process, but for most important biological reactions we can still do no more than speculate. Needless to say speculation on such matters is rife in the chemical literature; it is hoped that having read this introduction the reader will feel more competent to assess any ideas on these topics he may meet in more comprehensive treatments of the subject.

Finally it gives me pleasure to acknowledge my debt of gratitude to Drs. J. S. E. Holker and D. G. Buckley who read the manuscript and made many helpful suggestions which lead to its improvement; to Mrs. E. George who prepared an impeccable typescript for the printer; and most of all to my wife, Ruth, who bore with patience and fortitude many months of book widowhood.

Cambridge   J. S.
May 1977

Contents

1. An introduction to metabolism

THE CHEMICAL reactions of living systems, so long regarded as the exclusive preserve of the biochemist, have attracted increasing interest among organic and inorganic chemists in recent years; and those chemists who have entered the field as active investigators have found a rich harvest of fascinating chemical problems ripe for solution.

The aim of this book is to provide an introduction to the subject in the form of a chemical approach to metabolism. Since it will be assumed throughout that the reader knows little or no biochemistry, it is appropriate to begin with an explanation of what is meant by that term. Metabolism is the collective word for all the chemical reactions which take place in living systems. The most telling way to appreciate its meaning is to spend some time studying a metabolic pathways map. Charted on the map are all the more important reaction pathways whereby organic compounds (metabolites) are interconverted in living cells to produce the complex molecules of life on the one hand and the waste products of metabolism on the other.

A map will probably be available for reference in your laboratory or library, or one can be purchased very cheaply. It would be useful though not essential to have a map available for easy reference while reading this book.

Reaction to the map will vary from person to person. The complete novice will probably be reminded of one of those children's puzzles where one is required to trace a pathway through a maze from start to finish. However, this maze has extra complications, in that it has no obvious starting point, and exit points are equally hard to find; almost always when one gets to the outside of the maze an arrow inconveniently points the way back to the middle and usually one can trace a full circle to return to the starting point by a different route. When viewed in this way, as no more than an interconnected set of chemical reactions, the pathways map seems a certain prescription for chaotic muddle, and yet in practice the whole system operates in a precisely ordered manner. This order is imposed by the metabolic machinery of the living cell. Clearly, therefore, before we embark on a detailed consideration of the chemical basis of metabolic reactions, we need to consider the biological environment in which they operate.

The first point to make in this connection is that not all the pathways shown on the map will be in operation in every living cell. Many animals, man included, consume both carbohydrate and protein foods and therefore require the pathways to metabolize both types of compound. On the other hand a yeast cell, growing on glucose as the sole source of carbon, will use the pathway of glucose metabolism, but the pathways associated with the breakdown of proteins will not be needed and will not operate. Similarly the end-products of metabolism can vary from one cell or organism to another. For example, the main fate of glucose in man is oxidation to carbon dioxide and water, whereas in a yeast growing under anaerobic (oxygen-free) conditions the glucose is converted mainly to carbon dioxide and ethanol. Such differences in the pattern of metabolism (i.e. pathways in operation) can also occur within a given organism between the cells of one part and another. In man, for instance, the pattern of metabolism in a liver cell is very different from that in a brain cell. So the metabolic pathways map does not show a set of reactions which is in operation in every living cell at all times. Instead it presents a composite picture built up from pathways which take place in a wide range of living systems. Only the more important pathways are included and therefore while a given cell may not use some of the pathways shown on the map it may use other pathways which are not shown.

Fortunately, although the pattern of metabolism can vary markedly from one cell to another, the task of building up a composite picture of the metabolic pathways is considerably simplified by the fact that there is a remarkable constancy within the pathways wherever they operate. Thus glucose is oxidized to carbon dioxide and water in the cells of a vast range of widely different organisms including animals, plants, and microorganisms. The process follows the same pathway throughout the range even though the enzymes that catalyse individual steps may show significant variation in structure from one organism to another. A further simplifying feature comes to light when the pathway by which glucose is oxidized to carbon dioxide and water in a mammal is set alongside that by which glucose is converted to carbon dioxide and ethanol in yeast. Although it leads to a different final product, the pathway in yeast follows exactly the course as that in the mammal for most of the way. Therefore, in designing the map it is necessary to show only one pathway, that corresponding to mammalian metabolism, with a branch at the appropriate point to show how ethanol is formed in yeast.

The functions of metabolism

In principle we could now begin to trace our way through the maze by selecting a particular type of living cell for study. The starting point for our analysis of the pathways map would then be determined by the food stuff of the chosen cell and the exit point would correspond to the material excreted from this cell. However, if we are to understand fully the chemical basis of metabolism we need to do more than just trace the flow of material along the various metabolic pathways. We need to explain in addition how the cell benefits from the flow and this brings us to a consideration of the various functions of metabolism.

The metabolic pathways can be classified according to their function into two main categories which together encompass the great majority of the pathways shown on the map. These are the catabolic pathways (catabolism) and the anabolic pathways (anabolism). The immediately obvious difference between the two types of pathway lies in the nature of the chemical change which they bring about. Thus a catabolic pathway has the effect of breaking down its starting material into smaller molecules whereas an anabolic pathway results in the biosynthesis of a complex molecule from smaller precursors.

The function of the anabolic pathways is straightforward: they provide the means of synthesizing the complex molecules needed to build, maintain, and reproduce the living cell. The starting point for an anabolic pathway may be a compound taken in as a part of the food material of the cell: an amino acid for example. However, for many metabolic pathways the starting material is not present as such in the food, in which case it has to be produced by the metabolism of the cell. This brings us to one of the main functions of the catabolic pathways: they serve to degrade the primary carbon sources taken in as food to produce the precursors of biosynthesis. A second vital function of catabolism is the provision of chemical energy in a form suitable for powering the various energy-requiring operations of the cell or organism. A third function is the conversion of waste material to a chemical form suitable for excretion from the cell or organism. The first two functions are the ones which will concern us most and taking them into account one can see that the pathways of catabolism and anabolism are not independent but closely integrated: the catabolic pathways service those of anabolism by providing the starting materials for biosynthesis and also by providing the chemical energy which is necessary for the successful operation of most biosynthetic pathways.

The pathway of glucose catabolism

This interrelationship can best be illustrated by considering the function of a particular catabolic pathway. The pathway of glucose catabolism has been selected for this exercise because it takes place in organisms of all types and is unquestionably the most important of all the catabolic pathways. Thus it provides an impressive number of metabolites which also serve as starting materials for vital biosynthetic pathways. In addition it is beautifully adapted to provide the living cell with useful chemical energy, and thus the breakdown of glucose provides a major source of this vital commodity. In view of its importance the pathway of glucose catabolism is considered to be one of the vital 'central pathways' of metabolism, and it is not surprising that it is awarded the place of honour at the centre of the metabolic pathways map.

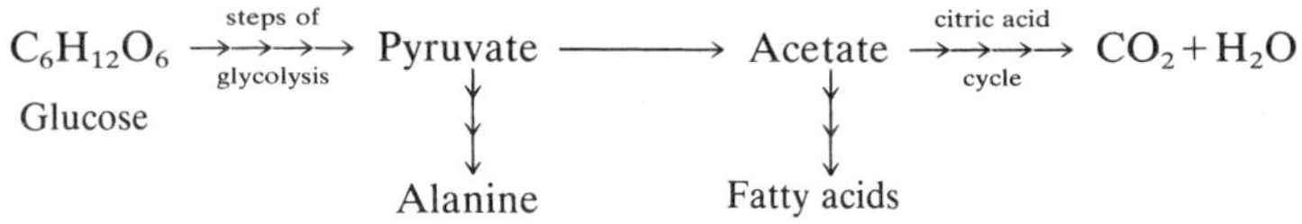

$$C_6H_{12}O_6 \xrightarrow[\text{glycolysis}]{\text{steps of}} \text{Pyruvate} \longrightarrow \text{Acetate} \xrightarrow[\text{cycle}]{\text{citric acid}} CO_2 + H_2O$$

Glucose

Alanine   Fatty acids

SCHEME 1.1

The pathway is shown in outline in Scheme 1.1. It is divided into two stages, one glycolysis, and the other the citric acid cycle, which operate in succession. The reason for this division will become clear when we consider the pathway in detail in Chapter 8. For the moment we shall concentrate on the fate of the two intermediates, pyruvate and acetate. The scheme indicates how one can serve as precursor for the biosynthesis of the amino acid alanine and the other as precursor of the fatty acids. Thus acetate is considered to be as the starting point for fatty acid biosynthesis. At first sight this may appear an arbitrary choice for one can trace a continuous pathway from glucose to fatty acids. What, then, is the basis for dividing the sequence into a catabolic stage (as far acetate) and then an anabolic stage (from acetate to the fatty acid)?

In fact the division can be justified on a number of grounds. Firstly, on chemical grounds, for the reaction sequence from glucose to acetate is definitely degradative in character, whereas from acetate to the fatty acids the sequence is unquestionably synthetic. Secondly, there are important biochemical grounds for the division, in that acetate is a branch point in the metabolic sequence from glucose to the fatty acids and therefore any mechanism for controlling the rate of fatty acid production must operate after that point if it is not to interfere with the rate of conversion of glucose to carbon dioxide and water. Thirdly, acetate can be generated in the cell from many compounds other than glucose so it is logical as well as convenient to consider the biosynthesis of fatty acids as if it started at that point. Finally the energetics of the pathway provide a further basis for making the division, for chemical energy is released in the conversion of glucose to acetate but a considerable input of energy is required in the conversion of acetate to fatty acids.

Bioenergetics

The energetics of metabolism will constitute a major theme of the following chapters and so it will provide a helpful background if at this

$$C_6H_{12}O_6 + 6O_2 \rightarrow 6CO_2 + 6H_2O$$

SCHEME 1.2

stage we examine in general terms how the chemical energy released in the course of glucose catabolism is harnessed for use in other spheres.

The overall chemical process is one of oxidation at the expense of molecular oxygen as indicated in Scheme 1.2. Surprisingly, however, oxygen does not react directly with any of the intermediates of glycolysis or the citric acid cycle. Instead the oxidative steps of the pathway are carried out by various coenzymes. (A coenzyme is a compound which acts in collaboration with an enzyme to bring about a metabolic reaction. Sometimes the role of the coenzyme is solely catalytic but frequently (as in the case under consideration) the coenzyme functions effectively as a reagent and is transformed as a consequence of the reaction into a different chemical form.) The general principles of how these coenzymes operate will be illustrated by examining the role of the one most frequently involved, namely the nicotinamide coenzyme, NAD^+. For the purpose of this outline treatment it is not necessary to know the structure of the coenzyme or the details of how it acts, but merely to accept that it can act as a dehydrogenating agent in a variety of metabolic reactions. In the process two hydrogens are abstracted from the substrate (which is therefore oxidized) and the coenzyme is reduced to its dihydro derivative, NADH. For example, one of the redox reactions of the citric acid cycle, the oxidation of malic acid to oxaloacetic acid, is shown in Scheme 1.3. The presentation of this reaction follows the standard biochemical convention. The double headed arrows signify that the reaction can take place readily in either direct ion in the living cell. In the pathway of glucose catabolism the direction of operation is from left to right. Note also that the reduction product of NAD^+ is shown as NADH rather than $NADH_2^+$. This is because the dihydro derivative of the coenzyme exists in the deprotonated form at pH 7. The reason for this will become clear when we meet the full structure. Following standard practice the proton will not be shown in subsequent reaction schemes of this type.

In the complete conversion of a molecule of glucose to carbon dioxide and water several molecules of the coenzyme are reduced in this way. In order to keep the process going on a continuous basis it is necessary that

$$HO_2C.CHOH.CH_2.CO_2H \rightleftharpoons HO_2C.CO.CH_2.CO_2H$$
$$NAD^{\oplus} \quad NADH + H^{\oplus}$$

SCHEME 1.3

the NADH be reoxidized to NAD^+ and this is where oxygen comes onto the scene. The reoxidation takes place at the expense of molecular oxygen in a specially organized enzymatic apparatus called the electron transport system as illustrated in Scheme 1.4. The coenzyme in its oxidized form is then ready to function once more as an oxidizing agent at one of the redox reactions of glucose catabolism in association with the appropriate enzyme. Thus the nicotinamide coenzyme functions effectively as a hydrogen carrier by shuttling backwards and forwards between the enzymes of glycolysis and the citric acid cycle on the one hand and the electron transport system on the other, and, although glucose is oxidized at the expense of molecular oxygen, the process takes place in a roundabout way.

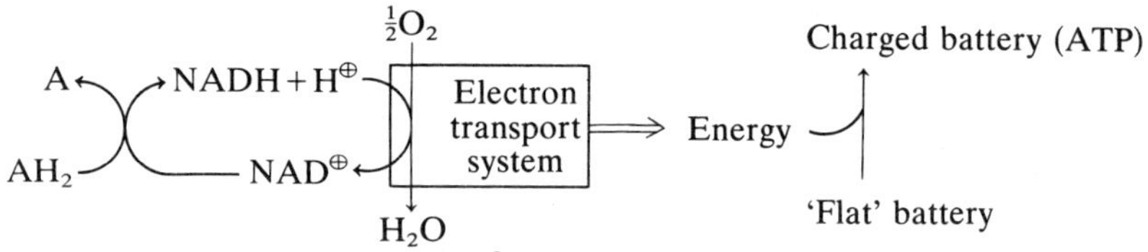

SCHEME 1.4

The chemical by-product of the reoxidation of NADH in the electron transport system is water but the really significant by-product from the metabolic point of view is the large amount of energy released ($220 \, \text{kJ mol}^{-1}$). The chemical energy is not just dissipated as heat but part is conserved for use elsewhere. To understand how this is achieved it is necessary to introduce a second coenzyme ATP. The structure and mode of operation of this compound will be covered in the next chapter; for the moment it is sufficient to picture it as a chemical battery which can be 'charged up' with energy at one point and then discharged to do useful work at another. In addition to bringing about the reoxidation of NADH the electron transport system has the remarkable ability to harness the energy liberated in the process to effect the regeneration of ATP as indicated in Scheme 1.4. Thus the electron transport system can be viewed as the power-house of the living cell in the sense that it 'burns' NADH as fuel and harnesses the resultant energy to recharge the chemical battery.

Needless to say, this simple treatment of the subject cannot tell the whole story, and to avoid confusion later two very important deficiencies should be mentioned. Firstly, NADH is not the only 'fuel' acceptable to the electron transport system: in one of the steps of the citric acid cycle succinic acid is dehydrogenated to fumaric acid; this process takes place directly in the electron transport system without the assistance of NADH and the resultant energy is harnessed for ATP production. Secondly, the electron transport system is not the sole means of harnessing the energy liberated in the course of glucose catabolism, for ATP generation takes place as an integral part of certain steps on the pathway.

Thirdly, to keep the energetics of metabolism in perspective, it should be remembered that glucose is not the only carbon source used for energy production in living cells; other food materials including fats and proteins are degraded in a similar way to produce NADH as fuel for the electron transport system. Finally we have to bear in mind that the original source of all the energy available to living organisms is the radiant energy of sunlight. This energy is harnessed by the photosynthetic apparatus of green plants to bring about the synthesis of carbohydrates such as glucose from carbon dioxide and water. So, viewed from the perspective of the biosphere as a whole, glucose is seen not as the starting point of metabolism but as an energy storage compound: having been synthesized in the plant kingdom as a means of storing the energy of sunlight, it is subsequently degraded to produce chemical energy, either in the cells of the plant which produced it or in the cells of another organism which has consumed the plant.

The scope of the chemical approach

This brief survey of metabolism is intended to set the scene for later chapters where key metabolic processes are considered in detail. Obviously, in treating the various reactions we shall be interested in the question of reaction mechanism. In addition, however, we shall need to consider the factors which govern the net direction of flow of material along metabolic pathways. Therefore, in the treatment of the chemical basis of individual reactions the question of equilibrium and free-energy change will loom large, because it is this aspect of chemical reactivity which governs the favourable direction of operation of the process under consideration.

The early chapters will deal with the energetics and mechanism of a selection of metabolic reactions one by one. Then in later chapters some of the more important metabolic pathways will be traced step by step to show how the individual reactions mesh together to produce a coherent and smooth running system.

Before closing this introduction it is desirable to mention certain other aspects of metabolism which will not be covered. The first is the problem of how the pathways are regulated, that is to say how the rate of operation of individual pathways is controlled. For example we have seen earlier that pyruvate (formed from glucose) can either be oxidized to carbon dioxide and water to provide energy, or it can be used in the biosynthesis of the amino acid alanine. It is essential for the smooth functioning of metabolism that the rate of operation of each pathway

should be capable of independent variation according to the requirements of the cell while both pathways are in operation. The way in which
this is achieved, by controlling the rate of reaction at a key step in each
reaction sequence (for example by varying the amount of enzyme
available to catalyse the reaction), is a crucial feature of metabolism.
Fortunately, although this is a serious omission in terms of biochemistry,
it will not vitiate the chemical approach to metabolism adopted in this
book. We shall be concerned with the chemical processes which pump
the materials along the pipeline; the control mechanisms functions
effectively as a valve and in this sense it is a completely independent
problem.

A second aspect of metabolism which we shall largely ignore is the
question of the intramolecular location of the enzymes. The interior of
the cell is not homogeneous, but is divided into sub-cellular compartments. For a full understanding of the controlled working of metabolism
it is essential to know where enzymes are located, and how metabolites
are transferred at the appropriate stage from one compartment to the
next. Again this is a question of organization rather than chemical
reactivity, and so, generally speaking, we shall only refer to the location
of an enzyme when it helps to explain the chemistry of the process under
consideration.

Finally, it has been decided with regret that there will not be room in
this short book to give a comprehensive treatment of the subject of
enzyme catalysis. The field is so vast it would need a complete separate
volume to do justice to this topic even at the introductory level. So in
spite of the fact that this is an aspect of metabolism which is actively
investigated by chemists as well as biochemists, the coverage in this book
will be restricted to reactions in which coenzymes are involved.

Even with these important omissions we are still left with a wide and
fascinating brief: the mechanism and energetics of metabolic reactions. It
is hoped that having read this book the reader will be stimulated to
explore these subjects in more depth and also to range more widely into
the equally fascinating biochemical aspects of metabolism which will not
have been covered.

2. ATP: the chemical battery

HAVING surveyed the general plan of metabolism we are now ready to consider how it is put into effect at the level of individual reactions, and we shall start with the role of ATP. This coenzyme was dubbed the chemical battery in Chapter 1, on account of its central role in the harnessing, distribution, and utilization of chemical energy. In this chapter we shall consider in more detail how the energy stored in the battery can be used to do useful work. In each of the examples chosen for illustration the energy is used to drive an energetically unfavourable chemical reaction. Thus the work in question is done in the chemical sense rather than in the more familiar mechanical sense.

The structure of ATP

The structure of ATP, adenosine triphosphate [1] is shown below. The compound is a nucleotide and is closely related in structure to one of the basic units of the genetic code. Three standard structural sub-units can be recognized as indicated in the diagram.

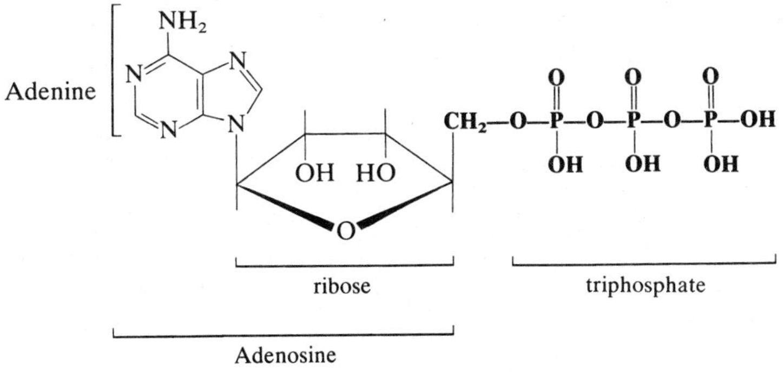

[1]

To the reader who is unfamiliar with biochemistry, the structure may appear alarmingly complex. Fortunately when we come to account for the metabolic reactions of ATP we need only consider the triphosphate residue. This is the only part of the molecule which undergoes structural alteration in the reactions which concern us; the rest of the molecule comes through unscathed. However, this does not mean that the structure of this non-operative part of the molecule is unimportant. Each of the biological reactions of ATP requires an enzyme to catalyse it, and the 'inert' residue plays an essential role in the process of binding the coenzyme to the enzyme. In simple terms the triphosphate is the working part of the 'tool' and the rest is in effect a 'handle' which can be recognized and gripped by the enzyme as a prelude to reaction. The importance of the handle can best be appreciated when the existence of other nucleotide coenzymes is taken into account. These compounds function in essentially the same way as ATP. They differ solely in the structure of the nitrogen heterocycle; for example, guanosine triphosphate (GTP) has a guanine residue [2] in place of the adenine unit of ATP. Even such a comparatively minor alteration in the structure of the handle is sufficient to ensure that the various coenzymes are not usually interchangeable, despite the fact that they have the same working part and carry out essentially equivalent reactions in their respective spheres of operation. Since ATP is by far the most important of these compounds it is the only one that will be treated in this account. In order to economize on space and also to make the meaning of the diagrams clearer the structure of the non-operative residue will be represented from now on simply by the symbol Ad as in the abbreviated structure [3] denoting ATP.

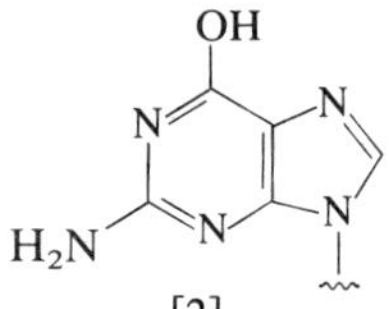

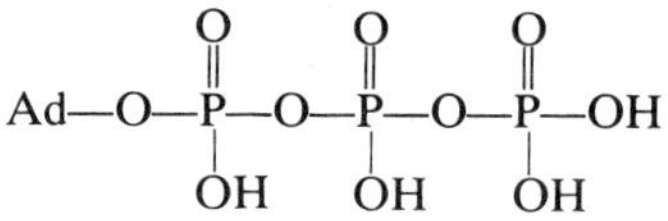

This is a good point to introduce some of the other abbreviations which will be used in this book when it is not necessary to specify the full structure of a compound. They are shown in Scheme 2.1. In each case the left-hand diagram shows the full structure and the right-hand one represents a more convenient condensed notation commonly used in biochemistry.

Free energy of hydrolysis of ATP

Given the structure of ATP we can now consider how the coenzyme functions as a chemical battery. The chemical energy stored in the molecule is released by cleavage of one of the bonds of the triphosphate residue. There are four possible sites of cleavage but in this chapter we shall consider only two, those marked by arrows in [4]. Scheme 2.2 shows the results of hydrolytic cleavage by reaction with water at these two positions. Cleavage at site (a) gives rise to adenosine monophosphate (AMP) and pyrophosphoric acid; cleavage at site (b) generates adenosine diphosphate (ADP) and phosphoric acid. Each reaction is

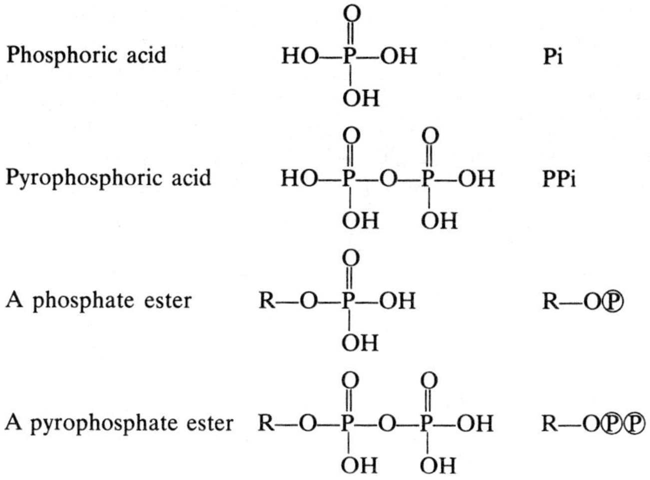

Phosphoric acid

$$\underset{\overset{|}{\text{OH}}}{\overset{\overset{\text{O}}{\|}}{\text{HO}-\text{P}-\text{OH}}}$$

Pi

Pyrophosphoric acid

$$\underset{\overset{|}{\text{OH}}\quad\overset{|}{\text{OH}}}{\overset{\overset{\text{O}}{\|}\quad\overset{\text{O}}{\|}}{\text{HO}-\text{P}-\text{O}-\text{P}-\text{OH}}}$$

PPi

A phosphate ester

$$\underset{\overset{|}{\text{OH}}}{\overset{\overset{\text{O}}{\|}}{\text{R}-\text{O}-\text{P}-\text{OH}}}$$

R—O℗

A pyrophosphate ester

$$\underset{\overset{|}{\text{OH}}\quad\overset{|}{\text{OH}}}{\overset{\overset{\text{O}}{\|}\quad\overset{\text{O}}{\|}}{\text{R}-\text{O}-\text{P}-\text{O}-\text{P}-\text{OH}}}$$

R—O℗℗

SCHEME 2.1

accompanied by the release of a relatively large amount of chemical energy ($\Delta G^{\ominus\prime} = -31$ kJ mol^{-1} for the hydrolysis of ATP to ADP and Pi), and accordingly the reactions go virtually to completion under physiological conditions. ($\Delta G^{\ominus\prime}$ represents the Gibbs function (free energy) change measured under standard conditions, but at a constant pH of 7. The role of the Gibbs function in chemistry is described in Smith's *Basic chemical thermodynamics*, OCS 28.) When ATP is cleaved by reaction with water the stored chemical energy is dissipated (mainly as heat). Consequently the chemical battery is discharged but without doing useful work; we shall meet reactions in which the energy is used to do work later in the chapter.

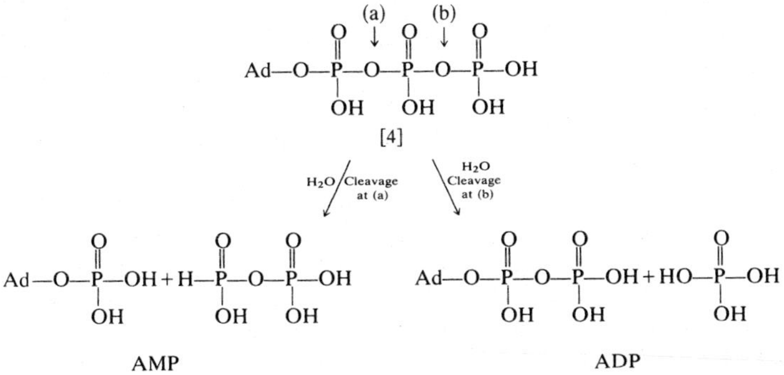

SCHEME 2.2

The ability of ATP to release so much chemical energy as a result of a simple chemical cleavage is essential to its function as an effective chemical battery. Consider, for example, the comparable cleavage of AMP to adenosine [5] and phosphoric acid as illustrated in Scheme 2.3. This process also liberates chemical energy but to a lesser extent than the cleavage of ATP. Therefore although AMP cleavage could in principle replace ATP cleavage in many of the metabolic reactions which depend on ATP for chemical energy, AMP would be a less effective form of chemical battery because it has relatively little energy in store.

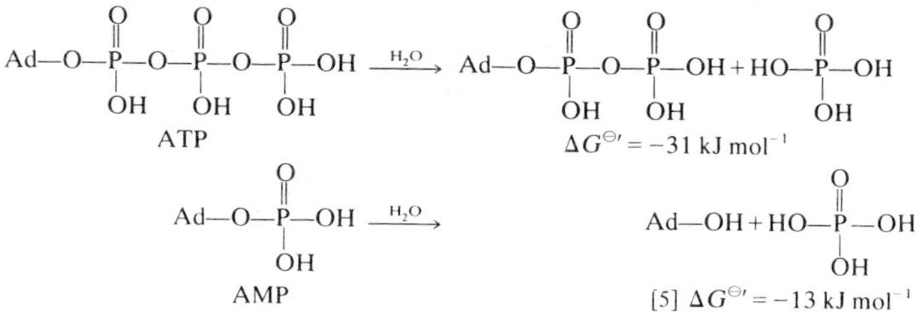

SCHEME 2.3

This is a good point to introduce the concept of 'energy-rich' and 'energy-poor' metabolites (alternative terms are 'high-energy' and 'low-energy'). An energy-rich compound is defined as one which can undergo a standard metabolic reaction (for example, a hydrolytic cleavage in the case of a derivative of phosphoric acid or a carboxylic acid) which is accompanied by a standard free-energy change equal to or greater than (in the negative sense) that associated with ATP hydrolysis to ADP. In other words the reaction in question releases an amount of chemical energy equal to or greater than that released by the chosen standard. Conversely a compound is considered to be energy-poor if it releases a lower amount of energy in an appropriate metabolic reaction. The choice of ATP hydrolysis as reference point is based on the central role it plays in the energetics of metabolism. Admittedly, this classification is essentially arbitrary but it does provide a helpful frame of reference to which we shall constantly refer in our analysis of the complex energetic inter-relationships which govern the direction of operation of various metabolic pathways.

Thus ATP can be considered to be an energy-rich compound. It must be emphasized that this classification does not imply that ATP has an exceptionally high free energy of formation (from its elements) or that it is explosive or exceptionally unstable. The term merely signifies that ATP can undergo a metabolic reaction (in this case a hydrolytic cleavage) that releases under standard conditions an amount of chemical energy equal to at least 31 kJ mol^{-1}.

The explanation of why the free energy of hydrolysis of ATP should be so high on the basis of its structure has been the subject of vigorous debate. The cause of the disagreement was the concept of an 'energy-rich' bond commonly designated by a 'squiggle' as indicated in [6]. The concept is well established, but it can be misleading and must be interpreted with caution. It must not be taken to imply that the chemical energy to be be released on hydrolysis is in some way packed into that particular bond, because free energy is an extensive property of the molecule as a whole. The significance of the squiggle is that it marks a point at which the molecule can react in a biological system to give products which have a much lower energy content than the starting material.

$$
\underset{\displaystyle [6]}{
Ad-O-\underset{\underset{OH}{|}}{\overset{\overset{O}{\|}}{P}}-O-\underset{\underset{OH}{|}}{\overset{\overset{O}{\|}}{P}}-O\sim\underset{\underset{OH}{|}}{\overset{\overset{O}{\|}}{P}}-OH
}
$$

In accounting for the relatively large amount of chemical energy released in the cleavage of ATP we shall continue to use as a basis for comparison the hydrolysis of AMP. In the context of the present discussion the essential difference between these compounds lies in the nature of the group that undergoes cleavage (see Scheme 2.3): in ATP this group is a phosphoric anydride, whereas in AMP it is a monoester of phosphoric acid. The greater thermodynamic reactivity of the phosphoric anhydride over the phosphate ester parallels the behaviour of the equivalent derivatives of the more familiar carboxylic acids. For example, acetic anhydride is thermodynamically more reactive than ethyl acetate, and thus liberates more energy on hydrolysis under standard conditions.

The relative reactivity of the anhydride and ester in carboxylic acid chemistry is usually explained in terms of electronic effects, and equivalent explanations can be advanced to account for the thermodynamic reactivity of the corresponding derivatives of phosphoric acid.

In all, three factors which might contribute to the greater reactivity of the anhydride will be considered. Firstly, the lone pair on the oxygen of the bond to be cleaved is delocalized with the neighbouring phosphoryl group. One can see from Scheme 2.4 that this delocalization is favourable in the ester [7], whereas it is inhibited in the anhydride [8] by an unfavourable electronic interaction with a second phosphoryl group. It should not be necessary to go into this explanation in any greater detail, but to emphasize the point, the equivalent derivatives of acetic acid, which should be familiar, are shown alongside in the scheme. As a result

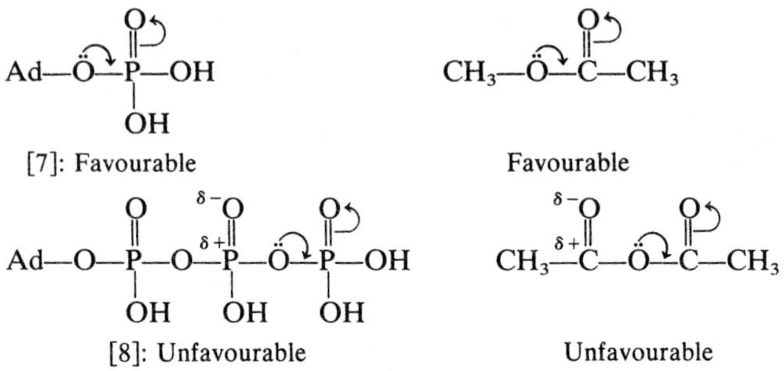

[7]: Favourable   Favourable

[8]: Unfavourable   Unfavourable

SCHEME 2.4

of this electronic effect the ester would be expected in each case to have a greater degree of stabilization than the anhydride and, in consequence, to have less free energy to lose on hydrolysis.

To appreciate the second factor it must be remembered that the hydrolyses under consideration take place at pH 7 and therefore the acidic hydroxyl groups in the starting materials are extensively ionized. In the case of the triphosphate this means that there are several negative charges in close proximity. This point is illustrated in Scheme 2.5, where, for emphasis, the structures of both the triphosphate and the monophosphate are shown in the completely ionized form. In the case of the triphosphate this gives rise to an unfavourable electrostatic interaction which is relieved by the hydrolysis. No such relief is gained in the case of the monophosphate, so the driving force for hydrolysis of the ester link should be less on this account also.

Finally, we have to take into account the fact that the hydrolysis in the living cell takes place at constant pH. Therefore the extra acidic hydroxyl groups generated in the products tend to be strongly ionized and this ionization increases the total amount of chemical energy released. In the hydrolysis of the phosphoric anhydride two extra acidic hydroxyl groups are generated compared with only one in the case of the ester, so this factor also helps the anhydride to hydrolyse more completely than the ester.

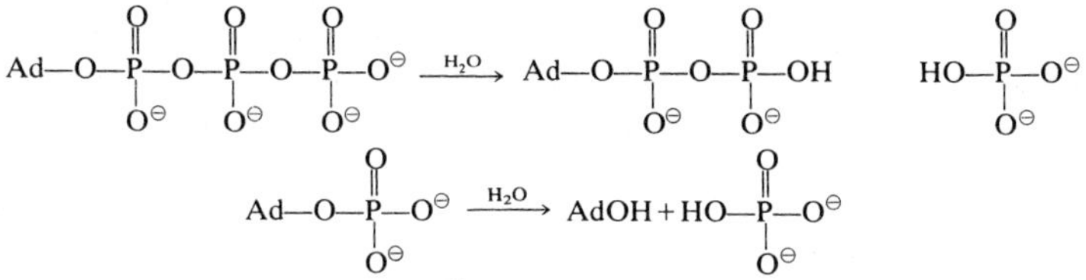

SCHEME 2.5

Though the validity of these explanations is open to question, the greater driving force for the hydrolysis of the phosphoric anhydride link in ATP compared with the monoester link in AMP is not in doubt for it is an absolutely reliable fact established by experimental measurement. It must be remembered, however, that the values quoted earlier for the standard free-energy change in these reactions were measured in free solution and may not hold exactly in the complex reaction medium of the living cell. Thus it will be apparent from the analysis of possible structural effects on reactivity, that the free energy of hydrolysis will greatly depend on the degree of ionization of the phosphate groups, and thus will vary with pH. There is a strong possibility that the pH will be considerably less than the neutral point in some compartments of the cell: for example, in the structure holding the electron transport system. A second environmental factor which may strongly influence the thermodynamic reactivity of ATP is the concentration of metal cations in the medium, because ATP and (to a lesser extent) ADP both chelate with such cations. In fact magnesium ion is essential to the biological activity of the coenzyme and the value quoted above for the standard free energy of hydrolysis of ATP refers to the magnesium complex. Nevertheless we have to accept these 'test-tube' measurements as the only ones available and, since it is probable that they are reasonably close to the true values obtaining in the cell, they will be used as the basis for our analysis of the energetics of metabolism.

Before closing this discussion of the chemical reactivity of ATP it is appropriate to comment on the kinetic stability of the coenzyme in free solution. In spite of the strong thermodynamic driving force for hydrolysis, the coenzyme is slow to react with water at pH 7, and this reflects the high energy of activation for chemical hydrolysis at this pH. This kinetic stability is essential for the effective functioning of the coenzyme: ATP would be useless as a chemical battery if it were susceptible to rapid non-enzymic hydrolysis during its transport from the site of its production to the site of its use, for such a process would result in wasteful dissipation of the stored chemical energy as heat. Instead ATP can move around the cell with the energy safely locked away until it is released to do useful work by the catalytic effect of an enzyme.

ATP and the performance of chemical work

The reactions shown in Scheme 2.6 are important metabolic transformations which, unfortunately, have large positive values of free-energy change in the direction indicated. In each case the process is driven against this adverse energy gradient with the assistance of ATP so that the chemical energy stored in the chemical battery is used to perform useful chemical work.

(1) Preparation of thioesters
$$RSH + R'CO_2H \longrightarrow R'COSR + H_2O$$
(2) Phosphorylation of alcohols
$$ROH + H_3PO_4 \longrightarrow R\!-\!O\!-\!\textcircled{P} + H_2O$$
(3) Carboxylation
$$CO_2 + CH_3.CO.CO_2H \longrightarrow HO_2C.CH_2.CO.CO_2H$$

SCHEME 2.6

We shall consider how this takes place by examining in detail the energetics of thioester formation. A full account of the metabolic functions of this type of compound will be given in Chapter 4. At this stage the only aspect of their biochemistry we need to know is that the standard free energy of hydrolysis of a thioester is large and negative ($\Delta G^{\ominus\prime} = -32$ kJ mol^{-1}). On this basis such compounds can be considered energy-rich and when they are allowed to reach equilibrium with an aqueous environment their hydrolysis is virtually complete. Conversely, when a carboxylic acid and a thiol are allowed to react in aqueous solution at pH 7 only a minute proportion of thioester is formed at equilibrium and therefore this direct approach is of no practical value as a chemical method of preparation. Similarly the direct reaction would be inefficient as a step of a metabolic pathway.

For the moment we shall treat the process as it operates in isolation. Under these conditions it only takes place to a useful extent if an external source of energy is provided to drive it up the energy hill. This is where the chemical energy stored in ATP can be put to good effect. If the coenzyme is added to the aqueous reaction mixture, together with the enzyme (or enzymes) appropriate to the particular carboxylic acid and thiol, a rapid net synthesis of thioester takes place (it is assumed, of course, that the reactants are metabolic intermediates and that the appropriate enzyme(s) are available; this is often the case and the process then provides a convenient method for the preparation of the particular thioester in the laboratory).

For every molecule of thioester produced in this enzyme-mediated reaction one molecule of ATP is hydrolysed to ADP. In effect, two potentially separate reactions become coupled, with the consequence that the chemical energy liberated in the cleavage of the ATP is not wasted as heat but is used instead to do useful chemical work in driving thioester formation. Since the values of the standard free energy of hydrolysis of the thioester and ATP are almost exactly equal (-31 and -32 kJ mol^{-1} respectively) the equilibrium constant of the coupled reaction is close to unity. Hence, starting with equimolar amounts of

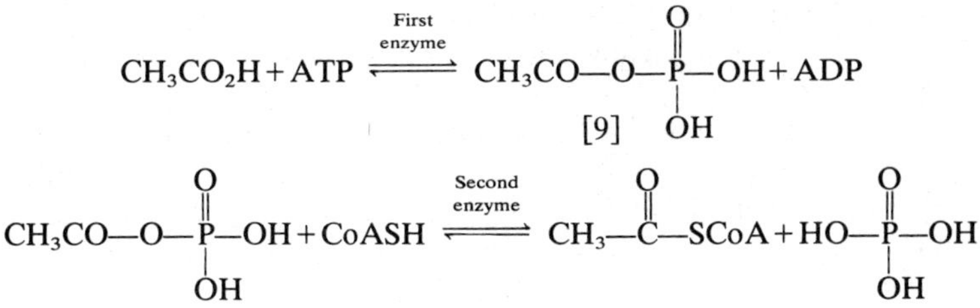

$$CH_3CO_2H + ATP \xrightleftharpoons[]{\text{First enzyme}} CH_3CO-O-\underset{\underset{OH}{|}}{\overset{\overset{O}{\|}}{P}}-OH + ADP$$

[9]

$$CH_3CO-O-\underset{\underset{OH}{|}}{\overset{\overset{O}{\|}}{P}}-OH + CoASH \xrightleftharpoons[]{\text{Second enzyme}} CH_3-\overset{\overset{O}{\|}}{C}-SCoA + HO-\underset{\underset{OH}{|}}{\overset{\overset{O}{\|}}{P}}-OH$$

SCHEME 2.7.

carboxylic acid, thiol, and ATP, approximately 50% of the starting materials are converted to products at equilibrium.

There are several reaction pathways by which this coupling is achieved in practice depending on the enzymes involved. They differ only in detail, however, so the general principles of their operation can be explained by examining how the process is carried out by an enzyme system of bacterial origin. In this case the carboxylic acid is acetic acid and the thiol is coenzyme A. The structure and biological role of this coenzyme will by treated in depth in Chapter 4. For the moment the structure will be represented in abbreviated form by CoASH (CoA is an abbreviation representing the complex 'handle' of the coenzyme, and SH denotes a thiol group which serves as the operative part). The product of the reaction is the coenzyme A ester of acetic acid, acetyl CoA.

The system under consideration (see Scheme 2.7) is unusual in that two separate enzymes are involved which operate in sequence. The first enzyme catalyses the reaction of ATP with acetic acid to form acetyl phosphate [9]. This intermediate is then released so that it can travel to the second enzyme on which it reacts with coenzyme A to form acetyl CoA. The overall effect is that for each molecule of thioester generated one molecule of ATP suffers hydrolysis, in this case to ADP and phosphate.

It is interesting to compare this reaction strategy with some of the standard methods adopted by organic chemists to overcome essentially the same problem, i.e. the preparation of an oxygen ester from a carboxylic acid and an alcohol. Usually, the direct reaction of an acid with an alcohol in equal amounts as shown in Scheme 2.8 does not give acceptable results because there is an appreciable amount of unreacted starting material at equilibrium. In laboratory practice this problem can be overcome in a number of ways. Thus, the equilibrium may be displaced by using a large excess of alcohol, or by removing the water as

$$RCO_2H + R'OH \rightleftharpoons RCO_2R' + H_2O$$

SCHEME 2.8

it is formed (for example by distillation). However, neither of these methods can be conveniently adapted for general use in the environment of a living cell.

The strategy adopted in the biological reaction does have a close parallel, however, in the standard laboratory approach which uses an acyl chloride as intermediate. A typical scheme of this type, using thionyl chloride as reagent, is summarized in Scheme 2.9, and to emphasize the parallel with the equivalent biological reaction both the chemical and biochemical reaction sequences are represented in the scheme according to the standard biochemical convention.

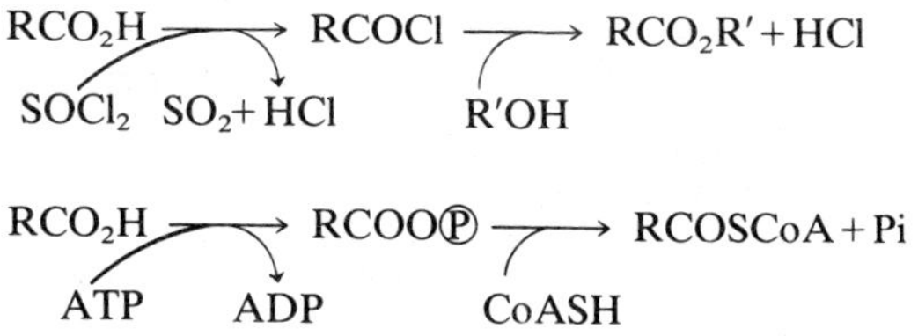

$$\text{RCO}_2\text{H} \longrightarrow \text{RCOCl} \longrightarrow \text{RCO}_2\text{R}' + \text{HCl}$$
$$\quad\quad \text{SOCl}_2 \quad \text{SO}_2 + \text{HCl} \quad\quad \text{R}'\text{OH}$$

$$\text{RCO}_2\text{H} \longrightarrow \text{RCOO}\textcircled{P} \longrightarrow \text{RCOSCoA} + \text{Pi}$$
$$\quad\quad \text{ATP} \quad \text{ADP} \quad\quad\quad \text{CoASH}$$

SCHEME 2.9

In the chemical reaction the acid is converted to a more reactive (energy-rich) derivative, the acyl chloride, while the thionyl chloride is hydrolysed to SO_2 and HCl. In this process the chemical energy released on hydrolytic cleavage of the thionyl chloride is used to drive the conversion of the carboxylic acid to its acid chloride. The reaction of the acid chloride with the alcohol in the next step releases much energy and goes effectively to completion Overall, the carboxylic acid is transformed to the ester in high yield, and the price to pay is the hydrolysis of one equivalent of thionyl chloride for each equivalent of acid undergoing the reaction.

Returning to the enzymic reaction, it will be apparent that the role of the acyl phosphate is equivalent to that of the acyl chloride. It is in fact a mixed anhydride of the carboxylic acid and phosphoric acid and its thermodynamic reactivity is reflected in a very high free energy of hydrolysis (to acetic acid and phosphoric acid. $\Delta G^{\ominus\prime} = -44 \text{ kJ mol}^{-1}$).

In this mode of coupling of the two biological reactions acetyl phosphate plays a crucial role by acting as a common intermediate. However, the formation of the acyl phosphate as intermediate is not the only way in which the coupling of these two reactions can be achieved. Thus the formation of acetyl CoA can be catalysed by a single enzyme, of wide distribution, called acetate thiokinase. The reaction scheme is clearly different from that discussed above because the ATP is hydrolysed to AMP and pyrophosphate not ADP and phosphate. A further significant difference is that acetyl phosphate is not formed as an enzyme-free intermediate. The acetic acid binds to the enzyme and the acyl group is not released until after the thioester has been formed. However, a multi-stage reaction sequence is still involved. In the first stage the acetic acid is converted by reaction with ATP to the acyl adenylate [10] and pyrophosphate. The acyl adenylate remains bound to the enzyme until it has reacted with coenzyme A. The products of this reaction, acetyl CoA and AMP, are then released.

$$\text{Ad—O—} \overset{\overset{\displaystyle O}{\parallel}}{\underset{\underset{\displaystyle OH}{|}}{P}} \text{—O—} \overset{\overset{\displaystyle O}{\parallel}}{C} \text{—CH}_3$$

[10]

While the details of this reaction sequence differ from that discussed earlier, the strategy is essentially the same from the thermodynamic point of view. The carboxylic acid is first converted into an energy-rich mixed anhydride which then drives the formation of the thioester. Thus thioester formation (and the attendant ATP hydrolysis) takes place by a roundabout route in which the water of the medium is no longer directly involved as a reagent and its status is reduced to that of an inert solvent (the elements of water needed to hydrolyse ATP are derived from the carboxylic acid and the thiol). The success of this strategy hinges on the fact that, with the benefit of enzymic catalysis, the rapid reactions of the biological pathway overwhelm the much slower direct chemical interconversion of the thioester and its hydrolysis products and so a state of pseudo-equilibrium is imposed on the system. Nevertheless, the chemical reaction still takes place independently of the enzymic process, albeit at a relatively slow rate. Hence, if the system is left for a long period of time, the thioester suffers gradual non-enzymic hydrolysis and eventually, the true chemical equilibrium is established in which virtually no thioester (or ATP) is present.

Factors determining the direction of flow

When in later chapters we consider metabolic pathways step by step it will become clear that coupled reactions such as those discussed above play a key role in determining the direction of flow of material. This applies particularly in the case of anabolic pathways which typically have an unfavourable inherent free-energy difference between the starting material(s) and final product(s), with the consequence that the overall transformation will not take place usefully in the required direction without assistance from an external energy source. This is where the energy stored in ATP can be usefully employed. Corresponding to each step of the pathway that is coupled to ATP cleavage there is a large negative (i.e. favourable) contribution to the net free-energy change associated with the formation of the final product. If sufficient steps of the pathway are modified in this way the overall free-energy change becomes favourable, and, as a result, the net direction of operation of the pathway lies in the direction of synthesis.

This train of thought will probably be unfamiliar to the average organic chemist who is accustomed to dealing with standard organic syntheses which are characteristically made up of discrete and thermodynamically independent steps. In contrast, the steps of a metabolic pathway are interconnected and the whole sequence is in effect one multi-stage reaction. It may be helpful therefore to consider an analogy in which the metabolic pathway is viewed as a continuous pipeline through which material flows from starting material to product. In the case of an energetically unfavourable pathway the pipeline runs up an energy hill and so the material has to be pumped in the required direction at the expense of an external energy source. In a sense, therefore, a coupled reaction can be regarded as a pumping stage on the pipeline.

While this analogy is fresh it is worth digressing briefly from the central theme to consider the wider problem of accounting for the direction of flow on metabolic pathways. Many pathways (usually catabolic) run down an energy hill in the desired direction, and consequently the required flow takes place without external assistance. Here the key steps can be regarded as waterfalls on the pipeline because they take place with a relatively large release of free energy and so play a major part in determining the direction of flow. Such steps are particularly interesting when, as sometimes happens, they are coupled to the formation of ATP, for then the energy released in the 'waterfall' is harnessed to recharge the chemical battery.

Though this analogy helps to explain the nature of the key steps it begs the question of what approach should be followed in analysing their thermodynamic basis. Generally speaking our approach will be that followed above in the treatment of thioester formation. Each reaction will be considered as though it takes place as an isolated equilibrium: in other words not subject to continuous supply of starting material and removal of product. The advantage of this somewhat artificial approach is that it allows the thermodynamic characteristics of the individual steps to be discussed in terms familiar to the average organic chemist. On this basis a 'pumping station' will be characteristically a transformation which is subjected in the context of a metabolic pathway to an external driving force so that its notional position of equilibrium will not be that expected on the basis of the inherent free-energy difference between the starting material and products, but will be displaced in favour of product formation. Conversely a transformation which is equivalent to a 'waterfall' will be characterized by an inherently favourable free-energy change, so that the notional position of equilibrium will lie strongly in favour of product formation without the assistance of an external driving force.

The full cycle of the chemical battery

At this stage it is a good idea to stand back and look at the role of ATP in thioester formation in a broader perspective. We saw in the opening chapter that ATP is formed as a consequence of the reactions of catabolism, for instance, in the electron transport system. The formation is merely the reversal of the hydrolysis—ADP is combined with phosphate to give ATP and water—and in the electron transport system the energy to drive this energetically unfavourable process is provided by the oxidation of NADH to NAD^+. The ATP thus formed joins the general pool of this metabolite from which it can be drawn as needed to drive energetically unfavourable reactions such as those we have considered. In these reactions ATP is usually hydrolysed to ADP and phosphate and the cycle is complete (see Scheme 2.10). So the analogy of ATP with a chemical battery is apt: the 'charged' form is ATP, while ADP and phosphate together represent a 'flat' form of the battery, and in essence the coenzyme serves as a medium for the transfer of energy from one part of the metabolic machine to another.

The same fundamental principles of operation govern the use of ATP to bring about the phosphorylation of an alcohol (reaction 2 of Scheme 2.6). The direct reaction is again characterized by an adverse free-energy change ($\Delta G^{\ominus\prime} = +13\,\text{kJ mol}^{-1}$). This thermodynamic barrier is overcome by drawing on the chemical energy released in catabolism as shown in Scheme 2.11. In this case the phosphate is not recycled but the role of ATP is still essentially that of a chemical battery.

In the two examples chosen for discussion we have seen how the energy stored in ATP can be used to perform work in the chemical sense

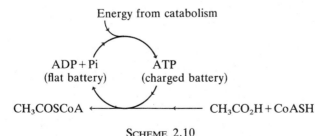

Energy from catabolism

ADP + Pi   ATP
(flat battery)   (charged battery)

$CH_3COSCoA \longleftarrow \qquad \longleftarrow CH_3CO_2H + CoASH$

SCHEME 2.10

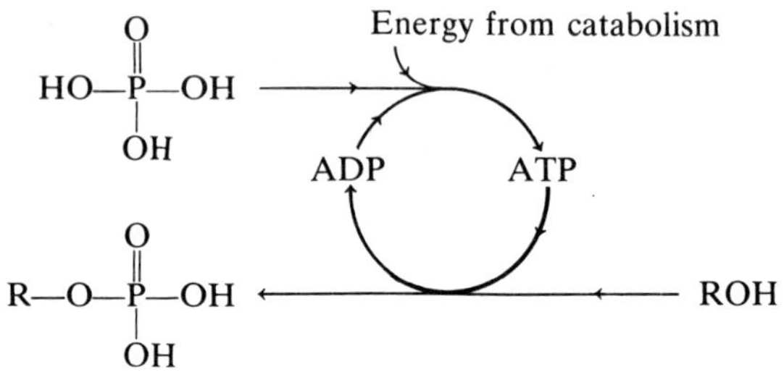

SCHEME 2.11.

by driving energetically unfavourable reactions. Further examples in which ATP functions in this sense will appear in later chapters. However, it must be remembered that energy is required to drive a vast range of different functions in living systems: to perform mechanical work in the muscle, to generate light in the firefly and electrical energy in nerve cells (or, more spectacularly, in the electric eel). ATP has a role to play in every case and one could devote the whole of this book to this single coenzyme and still not have room to do justice to its importance.

3. Phosphates, energy-rich and energy-poor

We now know that ATP can provide the energy to drive a thermodynamically unfavourable chemical transformation by undergoing cleavage at one of the anhydride bonds of the triphosphate group. In the two examples considered in the last chapter, thioester formation and the phosphorylation of an alcohol, the immediate consequence of the reaction of ATP was the conversion of the substrate (in an enzyme-mediated reaction the compound which is chemically transformed) to a phosphoryl derivative. This is the usual (though not universal) mode of operation of ATP and so it is not surprising to find a variety of different phosphoryl derivatives playing their part in the processes of metabolism.

In this chapter we shall examine the role of the following types of derivative: esters of phosphoric acid and pyrophosphoric acid, phosphoric anhydrides, and phosphoguanidines. These various derivatives play a vital part in the energetics of metabolism, and we shall see how the reactivity of their phosphoryl groups is nicely graded so that they can mesh together to serve the two-fold purpose of bioenergetics: the provision of chemical energy in the form of ATP on the one hand and the utilization of this energy on the other.

Phosphate and pyrophosphate esters of alcohols

One striking feature of phosphate metabolism is the frequency with which ATP is used to convert an alcohol to its phosphate ester as in Scheme 3.1. The formation of a phosphate ester uses ATP and thus depletes the energy reserves of the cell, so it is reasonable to suppose that the workings of metabolism benefit in some way from the transformation. In this section we shall study the fate of some phosphate and pyrophosphate esters formed in this way to try to discover what advantage can accrue from the process.

The pathway of terpene and steroid biosynthesis is an ideal case study because it relies heavily on phosphate ester chemistry, particularly in the early steps from mevalonate [11] to isopentenyl pyrophosphate [14]. A

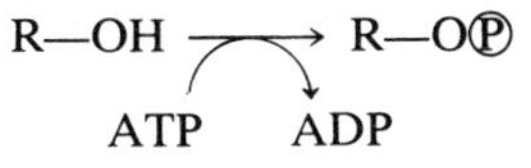

$$R—OH \longrightarrow R—O\text{\textcircled{P}}$$
$$\text{ATP} \quad \text{ADP}$$

SCHEME 3.1

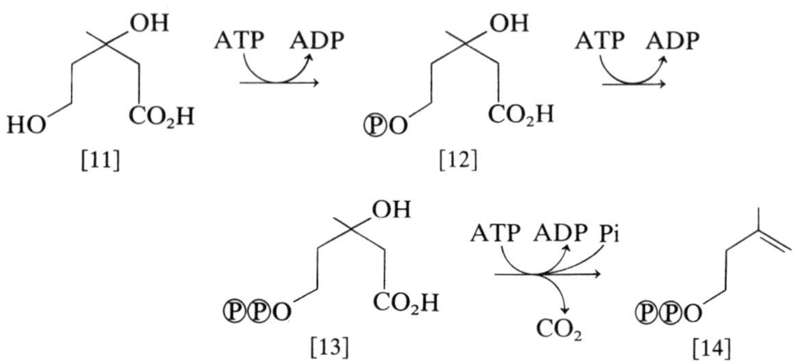

molecule of ATP is involved at each of the steps. In the overall conversion of [11] to [13] a pyrophosphate ester is generated at the expense of two molecules of ATP, but for the moment we shall concentrate on the role of ATP in the final step of the sequence, [13] to [14]. The mechanism of this reaction is not known, but it probably involves phosphorylation of the tertiary hydroxyl group prior to elimination and decarboxylation. A detailed mechanistic scheme, 3.2, is suggested for the process and it has been included to show the sort of way in which ATP might be expected to participate in the transformation. While the details of the mechanism are not known for certain, the proposed conversion of the hydroxyl group to a phosphate ester would have the advantage of facilitating the elimination step in the kinetic sense by generating a better leaving group.

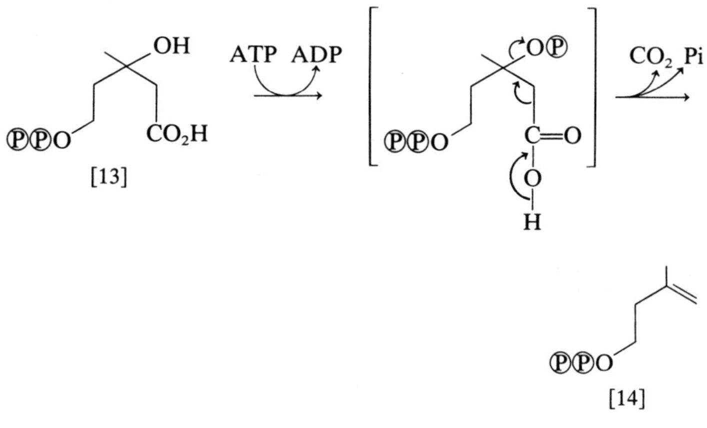

SCHEME 3.2

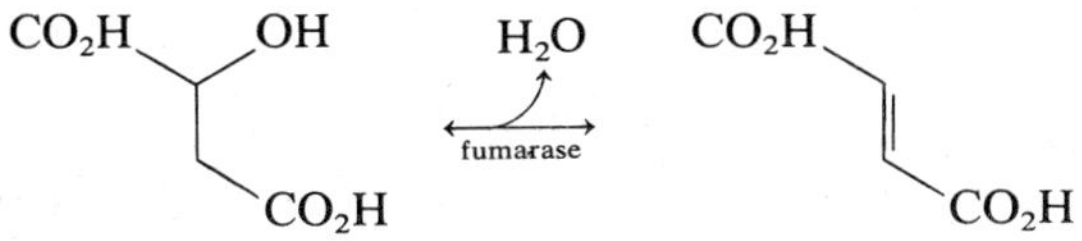

SCHEME 3.3

However, one needs to tread with caution at this point for there are many metabolic reactions in which a hydroxyl group undergoes elimination without prior conversion to a phosphate. For example, the interconversion shown in Scheme 3.3 is readily catalysed by the enzyme fumarase and we must therefore allow for the possibility that an enzyme could evolve which would catalyse the transformation of [13] to [14] without the expenditure of ATP. In that case must the hydrolysis of ATP in the existing elimination process be regarded as an entirely unnecessary expenditure of chemical energy? Probably not, because, whatever the advantage conferred on the process in the kinetic sense, the coupling of the elimination process to ATP hydrolysis will produce a definite benefit in the thermodynamic sense: the input of energy at this step will result in a favourable shift in the energy balance of the pathway as a whole.

In the earlier phosphorylation steps in the pathway, the primary hydroxyl group in [11] is converted to a pyrophosphate ester in [13]. To discover the advantage of this transformation one has to explore several steps further along the pathway. In the next step, part of the pool of isopentenyl pyrophosphate, [14], undergoes isomerization to form [15]. Compounds [14] and [15] then react as in Scheme 3.4, and the pyrophosphate group proves its worth by acting as a good leaving group in the enzyme-catalysed nucleophilic displacement. This use of the pyrophosphate ester, to facilitate displacement in the biological reaction, has an interesting parallel in the standard laboratory practice in which a hydroxyl group is converted to its tosylate ester prior to displacement.

The pathways of carbohydrate metabolism also rely heavily on the chemistry of the phosphate ester group. There is not room to give a comprehensive coverage so only one type of reaction will be considered at this stage, and that is the activation of the C-1 hydroxyl of glucose (or the equivalent hydroxyl group in other sugars) towards displacement in

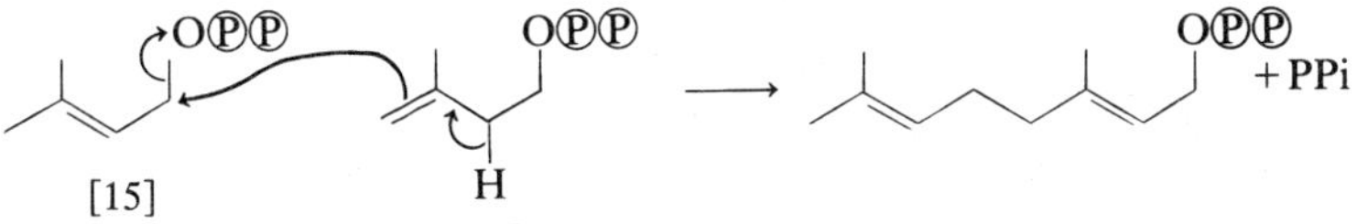

SCHEME 3.4

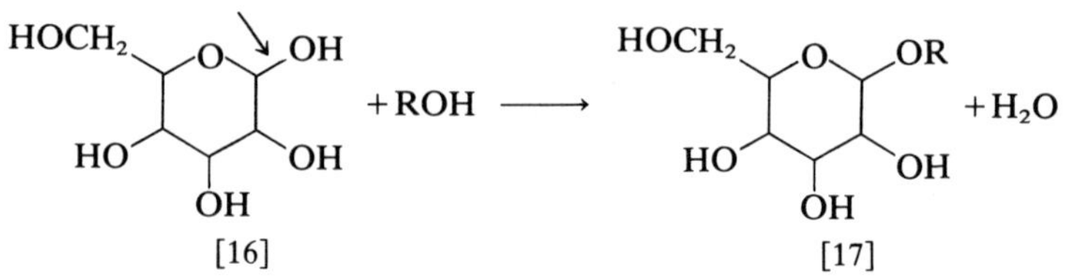

SCHEME 3.5

the biosynthesis of di-, oligo- and polysacchardides. The overall transformation in the reactions under consideration leads to the formation of an ether (glycosidic) link to a second carbohydrate molecule (ROH) as in Scheme 3.5. The bond which undergoes cleavage is indicated by an arrow in [16] and hence the reaction corresponds to displacement of OH by OR.

Enzymes capable of catalysing the direct interconversion of [16] and [17] do exist, but the direct process is of limited potential in the preparative sense as far as polysaccharide synthesis is concerned, because the normal position of equilibrium lies towards the hydrolysis products (the back reaction in Scheme 3.5). Therefore the biosynthesis of [17] from [16] is carried out by the indirect sequence of reactions shown in Scheme 3.6. In this sequence the C-1 hydroxyl is converted first to a phosphate and then to a pyrophosphate ester [18]. Note that in this compound the phosphoryl residue is ADP so that the product is a diester rather than a simple monoester of pyrophosphoric acid. Other

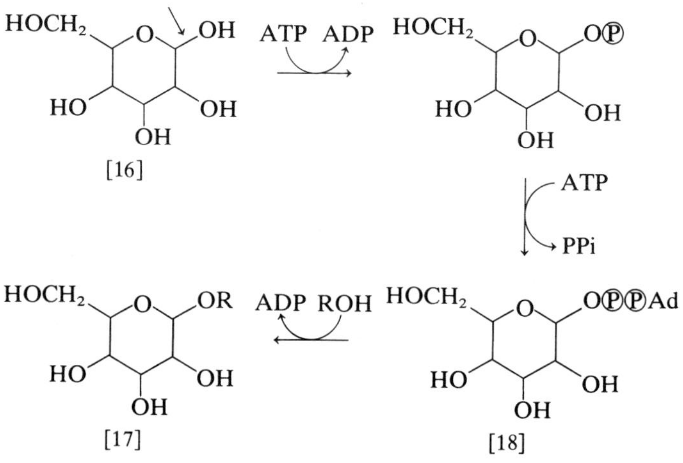

SCHEME 3.6

nucleotide coenzymes such as GTP can, and often do, serve an equivalent role depending on the particular biosynthetic pathway. However, as far as glucose is concerned the result is the same whatever the structure of the pyrophosphate residue may be: the C-1 hydroxyl is converted to a good leaving group for the final step, [18]→[17].

In view of what has been said above, we can be sure that the formation of the phosphate derivative is not essential in the kinetic sense for the displacement of the hydroxyl group at C-1 in the glucose: enzymes are known which catalyse the type of transformation represented by the interconversion of compounds [16] and [17] without the intermediacy of phosphate or pyrophosphate esters. In this case the advantage which accrues from forming the pyrophosphate ester is the conversion of glucose to the high-energy derivative [18] (free-energy release on hydrolysis: $\sim 30\,000\ kJ\,mol^{-1}$) so that the conversion of [18] to [17], releases free energy and the overall equilibrium now lies towards the desired product [17] rather than the starting material [16]. Overall, the sequence is beneficial in the preparative sense by overcoming the adverse free-energy difference between [17] and its hydrolysis products, and the price is paid by what amounts to the hydrolysis of two molecules of ATP to ADP.

Phosphoenolpyruvate

Phosphoenolpyruvate [20] is an intermediate in the catabolism of glucose and it plays a cardinal role from the point of view of bioenergetics. It is formed by dehydration of 2-phosphoglycerate [19] (note that the leaving group is not phosphorylated prior to elimination). The exceptional character of phosphoenolpyruvate is revealed in the next step in Scheme 3.7 where it carries out the phosphorylation of ADP to generate ATP and is itself converted to pyruvate. This reaction brings about a recharging of the chemical battery and it is one of the ways in which ATP is generated as a direct consequence of glucose catabolism, rather than indirectly in the electron transport system.

In this reaction a phosphate ester transfers its phosphate group to ADP and at first sight the process appears to run against the general pattern of phosphate chemistry which we have seen so far in this chapter.

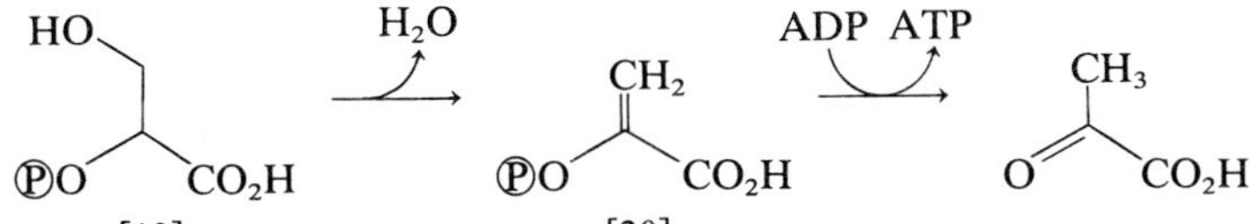

SCHEME 3.7

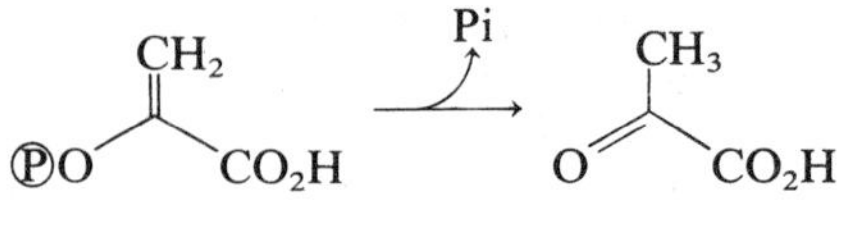

SCHEME 3.8

However, the reaction is understandable as soon as the free energy of hydrolysis of phosphoenolpyruvate is measured. This reaction, shown in Scheme 3.8, is accompanied by a free-energy release of no less than 55 kJ mol^{-1}, almost double that of ATP hydrolysis and no less than four times higher than that of an ordinary phosphate ester. On this basis phosphoenolpyruvate achieves the status of an energy-rich compound with spectacular ease and it is not surprising that the cleavage of its phosphate ester bond can drive the formation of the phosphoric anhydride group in ATP. Nevertheless the fundamental question remains to be answered: why should the enol phosphate residue in phosphoenolpyruvate release on hydrolysis approximately four times as much free energy as the phosphate ester of an alcoholic hydroxyl group?

One can find a precedent for this extraordinary reactivity of the enol phosphate in the general chemistry of the enol esters of carboxylic acids. For instance isopropenyl acetate [21] is commonly used as an acetylating agent in the preparation of the enol acetates of ketones as in Scheme 3.9. Acetic anhydride or acetyl chloride can also be used to carry out this reaction but the acetate ester of an ordinary alcohol, such as isopropyl alcohol, would not be effective.

The tendency of these enol esters to undergo transfer of the acyl or phosphoryl group in the reactions of Schemes 3.7, 3.8, and 3.9, is extraordinarily strong, and it reflects the thermodynamics of the keto-enol system produced on hydrolysis. Pyruvic acid exists almost completely in the keto form which indicates how unstable the enol is in comparison. In the enol ester the molecule is constrained to exist in the

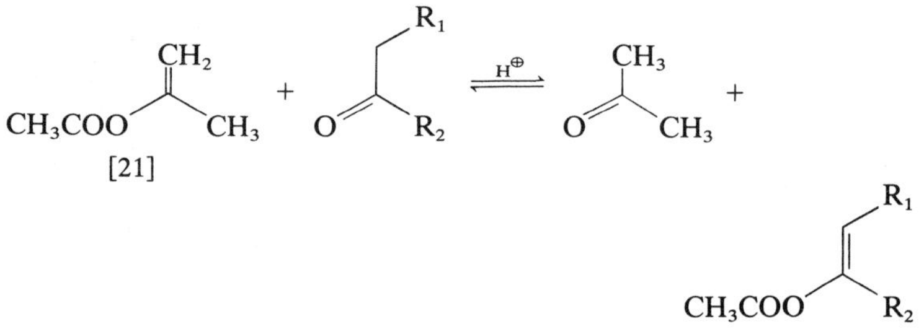

SCHEME 3.9

unfavourable enol form and therefore has more free energy to release on hydrolysis than would be expected on analogy with an ordinary ester.

As a consequence of the very great thermodynamic reactivity of phosphoenolpyruvate, the reaction with ADP as in Scheme 3.7 releases much free-energy, and it is therefore effectively irreversible in the preparative sense. Consequently, if pyruvate and ATP are allowed to react in the presence of the enzyme which catalyses the phosphoryl transfer, reaction will occur but virtually no phosphoenolpyruvate will be formed at equilibrium. Despite this thermodynamic barrier to the direct transformation of pyruvate to the enolpyruvate there is a metabolic pathway which achieves the conversion in an indirect way and it is worth considering it briefly because it illustrates an important aspect of bioenergetics.

The process is shown in Scheme 3.10 and it is a remarkably complicated reaction sequence to achieve what is essentially a very simple result. The basis of the reaction strategy, particularly the process of carboxylation followed by decarboxylation, will be discussed in detail in Chapter 10, and at this stage it is sufficient to note two points of general importance. Firstly, when the direct route between two metabolites is accompanied by a very large free-energy change a preparatively useful flow of materials will take place spontaneously in one direction only: the direction of free-energy release. The reverse transformation can only be achieved to a useful extent by a different and usually more roundabout process. This point is brought out in Scheme 3.11. Secondly, in driving the reversal, sufficient chemical energy has to be supplied to the system to pay the price of generating a thermodynamically less stable compound. In this respect it is significant that two molecules of ATP need to be hydrolysed to pay for the transformation of only one molecule of pyruvate to phosphoenolpyruvate. Finally, it must be emphasized once again that the enzymes which catalyse the two alternative pathways do not themselves influence the net direction of flow of material; the direction of flow is determined purely by the overall free-energy change inherent in the reactions themselves.

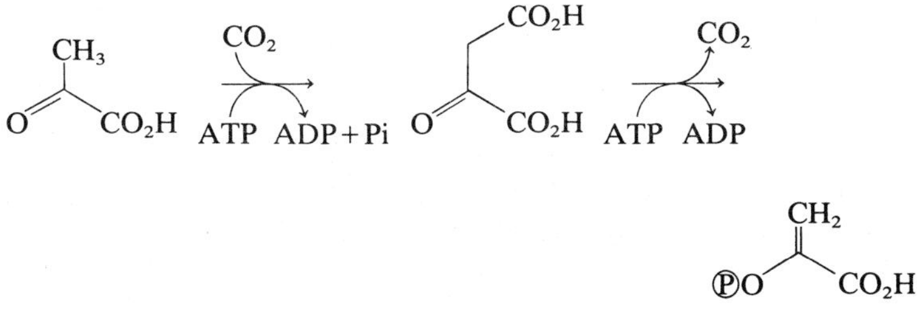

SCHEME 3.10

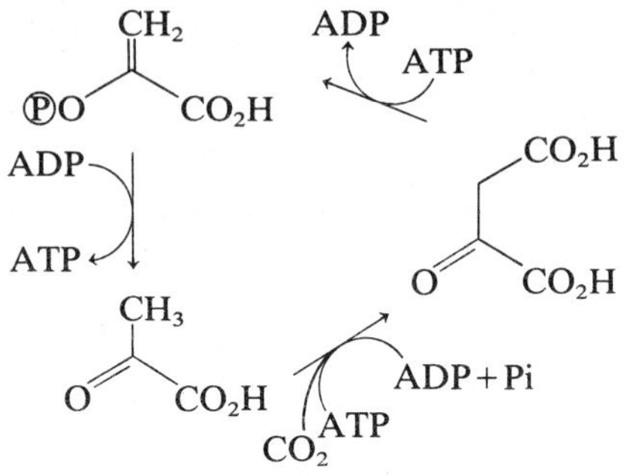

SCHEME 3.11

Before leaving this subject it is worth commenting on an alarming possibility raised by the reactions shown in Scheme 3.11. If this cycle were allowed to run wild by operating continuously in the anticlockwise direction all the ATP in the vicinity would be hydrolysed with no net gain to the cell. Presumably, this ruinous waste of chemical energy is avoided by ensuring that the two sets of enzymes operate independently in completely separate compartments, and this potential hazard illustrates the vital importance of the compartmentalization of the cell to the controlled operation of the metabolic machine.

Acyl phosphates

Acyl phosphates (the mixed anhydrides formed from a carboxylic acid and phophosphoric acid or other phosphoryl derivative) were introduced in the last chapter as intermediates in the preparation of acyl thioesters. This aspect of the biochemistry of acyl phosphate derivatives is extremely important but since it will be covered more fully in the next chapter it will not be considered in detail here.

The second major role of the acyl phosphate group is the generation of ATP. The free-energy release on hydrolysis falls in the range 45–55 kJ mol^{-1} depending on the structure. Even at the lower end of the range the value is approximately 50 per cent more than the corresponding figure for ATP, so it is not surprising that the formation of ATP from ADP can be driven by cleavage of an acyl phosphate. This process is illustrated here by the example of 1,3-diphosphoglycerate, [22], which undergoes cleavage of the acyl phosphate group as in Scheme 3.12, with concommittant formation of ATP from ADP. This reaction, like the equivalent reaction of phosphoenolpyruvate, is one of the steps of the pathway of glucose catabolism, so it represents a second example of how the chemical battery can be recharged without recourse to the electron transport system.

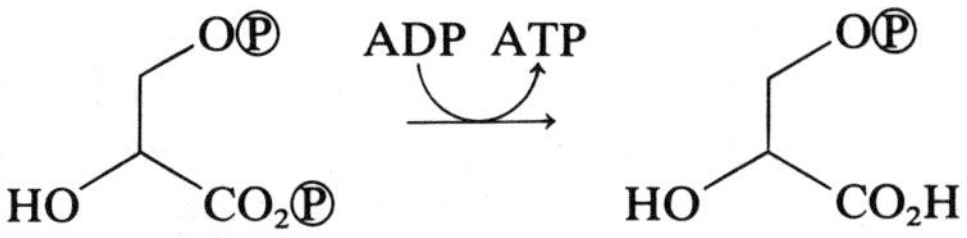

SCHEME 3.12

Phosphoguanidines

One of the aims of this survey of biologically active derivatives of phosphoric acid is to show how the thermodynamic reactivity of the phosphoryl group is profoundly dependent on its structural environment. In the structures we have considered so far the reacting group has been an ester or anhydride but the compound we are now to consider, phosphocreatine, [23], represents a class of compound in which the group undergoing cleavage is an amide of phophoric acid. Phosphocreatine releases sufficient free-energy on hydrolysis (38 kJ mol^{-1}) for it to be placed in the energy-rich class and its biological role as an energy storage compound in the muscle is based on this reactivity.

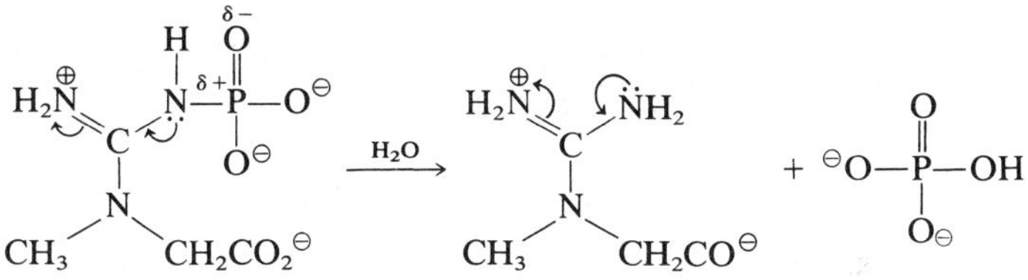

The surprising feature here is the large amount of free-energy released on hydrolysis of the amide link compared with that released by an ordinary ester of phosphoric acid (13 kJ mol^{-1}). Normally an amide is less reactive than the corresponding ester. One factor which will contribute to the unusually high thermodynamic reactivity of this particular amide is the peculiar structure of the guanidine residue. In the free amine [24], this residue has an extensively delocalized structure as shown, and the delocalization contributes to the overall stability of the hydrolysis product. In the phosphorylated compound this delocalization is inhibited by an unfavourable interaction with the phosphoryl dipole. As a result the energy difference between the amide and its hydrolysis products is greater than would otherwise be expected.

The phosphate group in bioenergetics: a summary

Before closing this chapter it would be helpful to summarize the principles which have been introduced so far and also to consider how the individual reactions fit into the wider framework of bioenergetics.

So far we have seen how the reactivity of the phosphoryl group is profoundly influenced by its structural environment and this gradation of reactivity is illustrated in diagrammatic form in Scheme 3.13. The diagram shows the four types of phosphoryl functional group which play a role in the bioenergetics of the central pathways of metabolism: the enol phosphate, the acyl phosphate, the phosphoric anhydride (e.g. ATP), and the simple phosphate ester. In each case the group is plotted alongside a typical (or actual) value for the free-energy of hydrolysis. An acyl thioester is plotted on the right of the diagram for comparison.

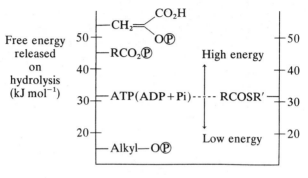

SCHEME 3.13

At this point we should recall that compounds are classified as energy-rich or energy-poor according to the value of the standard free-energy of hydrolysis relative to ATP. On this basis the top three phosphoryl compounds are placed in the energy-rich category and the ordinary phosphate ester is energy-poor. We are now in a position to appreciate the rationale behind this classification. A compound high on the list will have a strong tendency to undergo cleavage at the phosphoryl residue and will therefore be able to drive the formation of one lower down the list given a suitable enzyme. So phosphoenolpyruvate or an acyl phosphate can drive the formation of ATP to a useful extent as we saw in Schemes 3.7 and 3.12 respectively, but an ordinary phosphate ester is not sufficiently reactive. In turn ATP can drive the formation of an ordinary phosphate ester to a useful extent in a direct reaction as in Scheme 3.1 but it cannot similarly drive the formation of phosphoenol-pyruvate from pyruvate without resorting to an indirect multistage process which consumes more than one mole of ATP, as in Scheme 3.11.

Scheme 3.13 makes it clear that ATP is placed approximately midway on the range of reactivity of the phosphoryl derivatives and the point is often made that this is the ideal position for a compound which is to serve as the pivot for the interconversion of the different compounds in the series. Thus on the one hand ATP is sufficiently high on the scale to be capable of doing a useful job in driving many important metabolic processes which rely on the formation of an ordinary phosphate ester, but on the other hand it is not so high that it cannot be readily generated itself at the expense of the higher energy phosphates produced in catabolism.

Thus ATP is placed in a very strategic position with respect to other biologically important phosphates. Nevertheless it is arguable that its position in relation to that of an acyl thioester is even more significant but we will not pursue that train of thought any further at this stage, for risk of stealing the thunder of the next chapter.

4. Acyl thioesters and coenzyme A

AFTER two chapters devoted to the part played by the phosphate group in the energetics of metabolism we are now ready to consider the role of the carboxyl group and its derivatives. The progression is a natural one because the organization and successful operation of many aspects of metabolism depend to a considerable extent on the interaction of these two types of functional group.

Most readers will be already acquainted with a wide range of acyl derivatives, because the chemistry of the compounds in this series is one of the cornerstones of organic chemistry. Their importance is reflected in the numerous synthetic processes which hinge upon the reactivity of any acyl group of one type or another and it will become apparent that the acyl group plays an equally important part in the chemical reactions of metabolism. However, there is a very striking difference between the chemistry of the acyl group in the test tube and that in the cell: in contrast to the numerous derivatives employed by the organic chemist, the acyl chloride, anhydride, ester, amide, and azide to name but a few, the cell relies on just one key derivative, the thioester, to serve as the reactive acyl derivative in the majority of its reactions. Admittedly, other derivatives are employed but they have a very restricted role. For example, various acyl phosphates have already been discussed in earlier chapters. However, their function is to serve as reactive intermediate in the interconversion of acyl derivatives and the process has already been covered adequately. We shall see later in this chapter that in the formation of the amide bonds of proteins, the carboxyl of the amino acid is activated by conversion to the oxygen ester rather than the thioester. However, apart from a few exceptions of this type, the thioester is paramount in the metabolic reactions of the acyl group and the versatility of this functional group is one of the remarkable features of the chemistry of living systems.

Nature of the thiol residue

The commonest type of thioester is that based on coenzyme A. The structure of this coenzyme will be abbreviated to CoASH in line with standard biochemical practice but for interest the full structure is shown [25]. As far as is known, only the thiol group plays a direct role in the metabolic reactions of the coenzyme. The rest of the structure serves as a handle in the process of enzyme recognition and so we need not consider it any further, apart from noting that it incorporates two structural

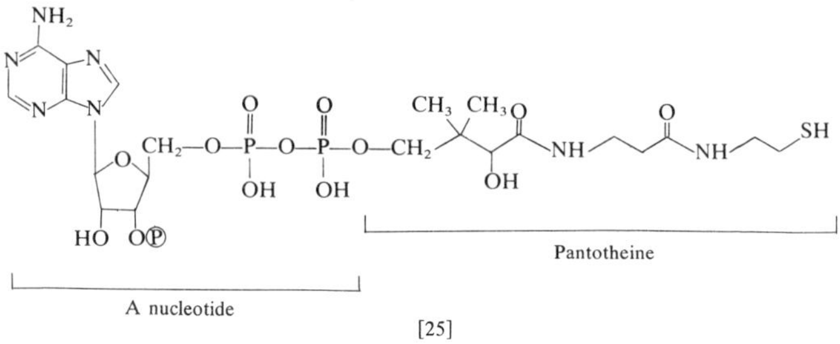

Pantotheine

A nucleotide

[25]

residues which occur in other coenzymes and catalytic groups, namely a nucleotide unit (almost identical with ADP), and a unit of pantotheine.

A thioester based on coenzyme A has the important advantage that once formed it can dissociate from the enzyme and travel to another to undergo further reaction. In this way the coenzyme serves as a reagent and vehicle for numerous carboxylic acids and an exceptionally large number of enzymes have developed the capacity to grip its handle.

A separate class of acyl thioester can be distinguished in which the thiol residue is an integral part of the enzyme on which the thioester reaction is to take place. In this case the thiol group may be that of a cysteine residue built into the protein chain of the enzyme in the normal way, as in [26]. However, in at least two examples of this type a specially adapted thiol residue is involved. For example, one of the enzymes of fatty acid synthesis incorportates into its structure a pantotheine unit (see [25]) and in the next chapter we shall meet acyl thioesters based on another specialized thiol residue, lipoic acid. Obviously, when the thiol group is part of the enzyme, the thioester has to be cleaved prior to release of the acyl residue and this represents an important difference in behaviour compared with that of thioesters based on coenzyme A. However, apart from this difference the two types of ester undergo essentially equivalent reactions.

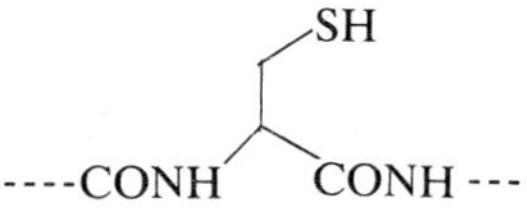

----CONH⁀CONH---

[26]

Methods of formation of thioesters

(1) *Esterification of a carboxyl group*

This reaction (Scheme 4.1) in which the process of ester formation is driven by ATP has already been discussed adequately.

$$RCO_2H + R'SH \xrightleftharpoons[\underset{ATP}{}]{\underset{ADP + Pi}{}} RCOSR'$$

SCHEME 4.1

(2) *Oxidative decarboxylation of a keto acid*

There are two examples of this type of reaction on the pathway of glucose catabolism. One of them, the oxidative decarboxylation of pyruvic acid, is illustrated in Scheme 4.2, and the process will be discussed in detail in the next chapter. This reaction, like the one above, leads to a net synthesis of thioester.

$$CH_3COCO_2H \xrightarrow[\underset{CoASH}{}]{decarboxylation} CH_3COSoA + CO_2$$

SCHEME 4.2

(3) *Exchange of the thiol residue*

In this reaction the thiol residue of a thioester is displaced by a second thiol group. The process provides an important method for the generation of enzyme-bound thioesters, as in Scheme 4.3, and the reaction frequently operates in the reverse direction to release an acyl group as the coenzyme A ester after completion of the desired transformation.

$$RCOSCoA + HS—Enzyme \rightleftharpoons RCOS—Enzyme + CoASH$$

SCHEME 4.3

(4) *Exchange of the acyl residue*

In this reaction the acyl group of a given thioester is replaced by another as in Scheme 4.4. The reaction provides an important method for the conversion of a given acid to its coenzyme A ester, at the expense effectively of the hydrolysis of the coenzyme A ester of a second acid. Therefore this reaction, like the preceeding one, does not lead to a net synthesis of thioester but merely exchanges one ester for another.

$$RCOSCoA + R'CO_2H \rightleftharpoons RCO_2H + R'COSCoA$$

SCHEME 4.4

Reactions of thioesters

In discussing the reactions of thioesters it is helpful to adopt a mechanistic approach. In each case the mechanism suggested for the biological reaction will be based on what would be expected for the equivalent chemical reaction. The justification for treating enzymic reactions in this way is that it helps to relate them to the more familiar reactions of organic chemistry and this policy will be adopted generally throughout the book. In discussing a particular enzyme any experimental evidence on the mechanism of action will be taken into account but the reader should always bear in mind that the actual mechanism will almost certainly be more complicated than that given, and that for a given type of reaction the mechanism may well vary in detail from one enzyme to another.

(1) *Nucleophilic displacement at the acyl group*

In this type of reaction the thiol group is displaced and in the following schemes the mechanism is portrayed as a nucleophilic addition to the carbonyl group followed by elimination of the thiol residue.

(*a*) *Displacement by a second thiol residue.* This reaction has already been mentioned as one of the methods of formation of thioesters. In Scheme 4.5 the mechanism is illustrated by the transfer of an acyl group from the thiol of coenzyme A to an enzyme-bound thiol, denoted by Enz-SH.

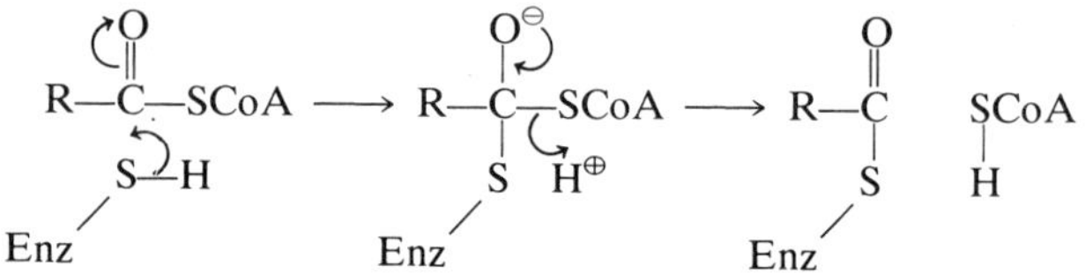

SCHEME 4.5

(*b*) *Hydrolysis coupled to ATP formation.* The simple hydrolysis of a thioester presumably follows essentially the same mechanism as that in Scheme 4.5, but with a molecule of water (or a hydroxide ion) taking the place of Enz-SH. However, a much more important reaction is that in which hydrolytic cleavage is accompanied by the formation of ATP. Normally, this transformation takes place via an intermediate mixed anhydride formed between the carboxylic acid and a phosphoryl residue which may be phosphoric acid itself or the terminal phosphate group of ADP. The process is illustrated here by an example of the former type in which acetyl CoA is converted to acetyl phosphate. The first step involves nucleophilic displacement of the thiol residue by phosphate as in Scheme 4.6. In the next step, shown in Scheme 4.7, the terminal phosphate of ADP carries out a nucleophilic displacement at the phosphoryl group of the mixed anhydride to generate ATP. The carboxylate anion is liberated in the last step, and so the thioester is converted indirectly to its hydrolysis products as a consequence of the overall transformation.

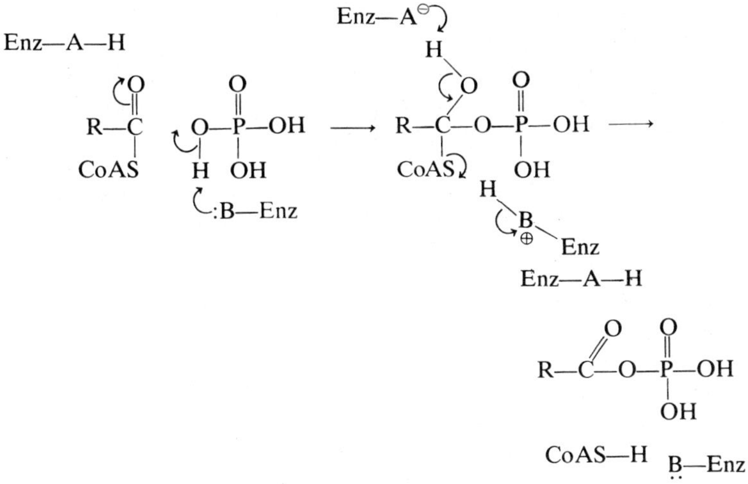

SCHEME 4.6

Note that the mechanism proposed in Scheme 4.6 invokes in the addition step a combination of acid catalysis (by the acidic group, AH, of the enzyme) and base catalysis (by the base B), followed by a complementary pattern of catalysis in the elimination step. This elaboration of the simplest possible representation of the mechanism is purely speculative and it is given to show how the enzyme might catalyse the reaction steps by having the appropriate catalytic groups in the correct orientation. Generally speaking, however, reactions will be portrayed

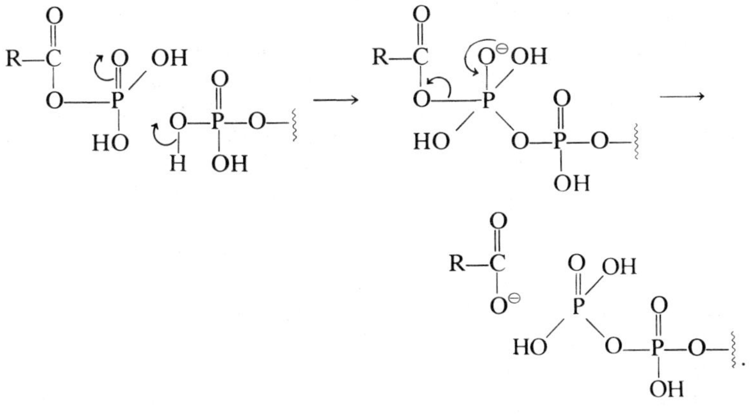

SCHEME 4.7

from now on in the simplest possible way to avoid unnecessary clutter in the diagrams.

Other functional groups which displace the thiol in an equivalent way include the amino group (for example in the formation of N-acetyl glutamate), the alcoholic hydroxyl group (acetyl choline formation), and hydride or its equivalent (to generate an aldehyde). In this series of reactions it will be apparent that the thiol ester plays a role equivalent to that of the acyl chloride or anhydride in organic chemistry.

(2) Conjugate addition

α,β-Unsaturated thioesters can undergo nucleophilic addition to the alkene bond as shown in Scheme 4.8. This type of reaction is not unique to the thioester derivative but can take place on the free acid as we saw earlier in Scheme 3.3. The proposed mechanism invokes the activating effect of the conjugated carbonyl group and it is significant that this type of hydration (and dehydration in the reverse direction) is characteristic of compounds in which a double bond is conjugated with the carbonyl group of one of the following functional groups: an acyl ester, a ketone, or an aldehyde.

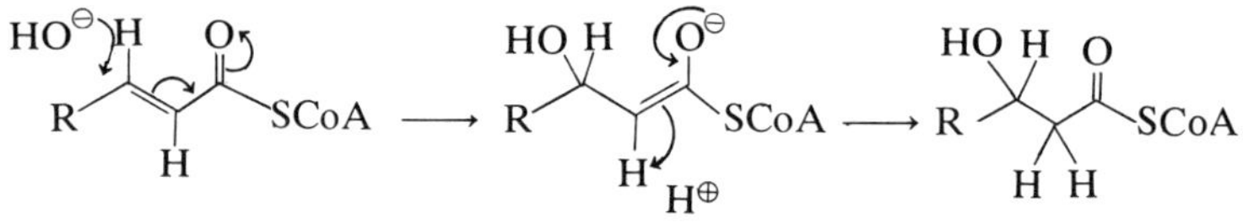

SCHEME 4.8

(3) Reaction at the α-carbon

In this class of reaction one of the hydrogens on the carbon adjacent to the acyl group is replaced by a new carbon-carbon bond. It is assumed that in the process the enolate (or possibly the enol) is generated as an intermediate, which then attacks a second molecule at its carbonyl group, typically that of an acyl ester or ketone. Synthetic reactions of this type occur frequently on the central pathways of metabolism.

(a) Attack on an acyl thioester: acetoacetate formation. In this type of reaction one thioester reacts in the enolate form and a second in the acyl form, and, as well as showing an enolate reaction, it represents another type of displacement at the acyl group, in this case by a carbon nucleophile. The reaction chosen to illustrate the process in Scheme 4.9 has a very close analogy in the Claisen condensation of ethyl acetate to form ethyl acetoacetate.

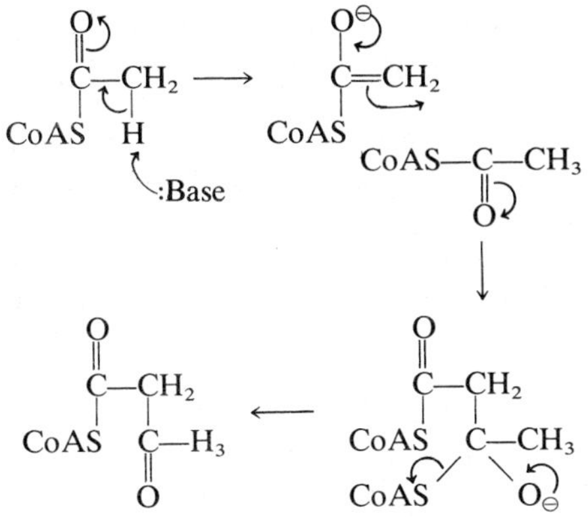

SCHEME 4.9

(b) *Attack on a ketone: citrate synthesis.* This reaction (an aldol condensation) takes place in one of the steps of the citric acid cycle. In the mechanistic Scheme 4.10 the nature of the thiol is not specified because although it is known that acetyl CoA is the substrate taken on to the enzyme there is evidence that the acyl group is transferred to an enzyme-bound thiol at some stage in the sequence of reactions. It is interesting to note that in this case the thioester is hydrolysed prior to release of the product. Presumably the hydrolysis releases free energy and so helps to drive the reaction in the desired direction.

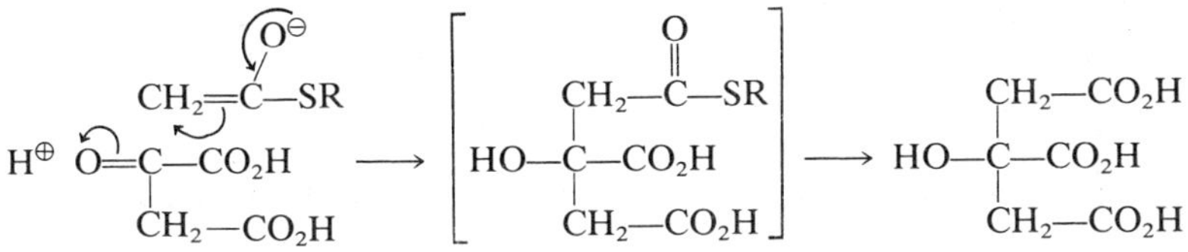

SCHEME 4.10

Thioesters versus oxygen esters as reactive intermediates in metabolism

The point has already been made in introducing the biological reactions of the acyl group that the thioester is employed almost universally as the reactive derivative and that this is in marked contrast to the usual practice of the organic chemist who uses a range of derivatives in carrying out the equivalent chemical reactions, selecting for each reaction the particular derivative of optimal reactivity. The list includes acyl chlorides, anhydrides, esters (oxygen), and, less frequently, azides and cyanides. Given that the reaction medium of the cell is aqueous, one can understand why the use of acyl chlorides and anhydrides would not be

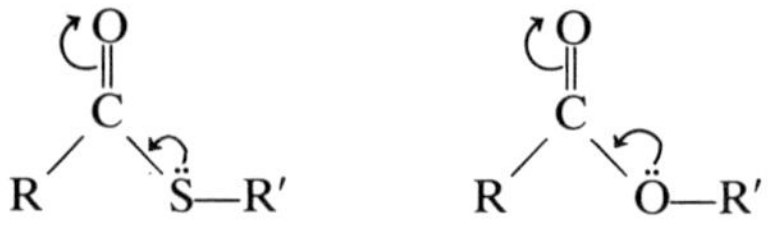

$$\text{SCHEME } 4.11$$

viable, but it is reasonable to ask why thioesters are dominant and oxygen esters almost completely absent as intermediates on the central metabolic pathways.

This brings us to the comparison which is often made in principle between the relative merits of the two types of ester as intermediates in the context of the metabolic pathways, and it is often suggested that the thioester would have the advantage of being more reactive because of the relative degree of delocalization in the two systems as shown in Scheme 4.11. Sulphur is much less effective at this type of delocalization than oxygen, and on this basis it has been proposed that the electrophilic reactivity of the carbonyl group of a thioester would be almost as high as that of a ketone in which this type of electronic effect is completely absent.

This assessment of the relative reactivity of the acyl group in the two types of ester has been supported by chemical investigation. Firstly, in a comparison of the two β-keto esters, [27] and [28], the central methylene of the thioester was found to be more acidic than that of the oxygen ester; in fact it was almost as acidic as that of the keto analogue [29]. The degree of acidity reflects the ability of the carbonyl groups to delocalize the negative charge in the carbanion and it is clear from the result that the reactivity of the thioester is closer to that of the ketone than that of the oxygen ester in this respect.

Secondly, chemical studies on the relative rates of nucleophilic displacement at the acyl group have shown that the thioester is usually

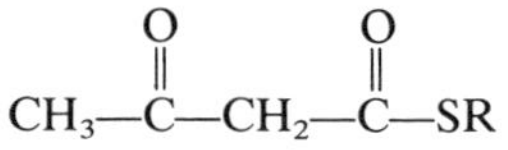

$$CH_3-\overset{\overset{\displaystyle O}{\|}}{C}-CH_2-\overset{\overset{\displaystyle O}{\|}}{C}-SR \qquad pK_a = 8 \cdot 5$$
$$[27]$$

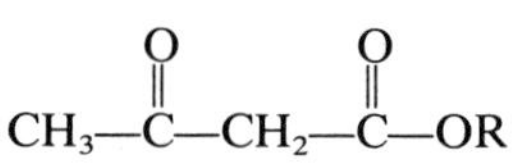

$$CH_3-\overset{\overset{\displaystyle O}{\|}}{C}-CH_2-\overset{\overset{\displaystyle O}{\|}}{C}-OR \qquad pK_a = 10 \cdot 5$$
$$[28]$$

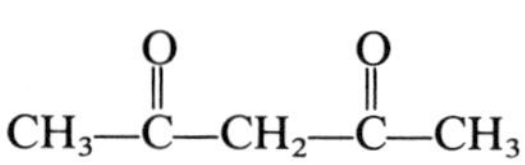

$$CH_3-\overset{\overset{\displaystyle O}{\|}}{C}-CH_2-\overset{\overset{\displaystyle O}{\|}}{C}-CH_3 \qquad pK_a = 8 \cdot 3$$
$$[29]$$

more reactive in this sense also. For example, in the transformation shown in Scheme 4.12 the thioester reacts much more rapidly than the oxygen ester. However, at this point it is necessary to enter a note of caution because the two types of ester were found to hydrolyse at comparable rates in the corresponding reaction with hydroxide ion. Presumably this result reflects the second effect that the sulphur atom may have on the overall rate of nucleophilic displacement: the carbon-sulphur bond is stronger than the carbon-oxygen bond and so will break less readily in the elimination step. Apparently this second effect makes its presence felt in the reaction with hydroxide and so cancels the greater reactivity of the acyl group in the first step. This result illustrates the danger of attempting to predict the overall rate of a multi-stage reaction on the basis of an effect which influences a particular step, which may or may not be rate-determining, and brings home the need for caution in attributing the dominant position of the thioester in metabolism to its potentially greater reactivity in the kinetic sense.

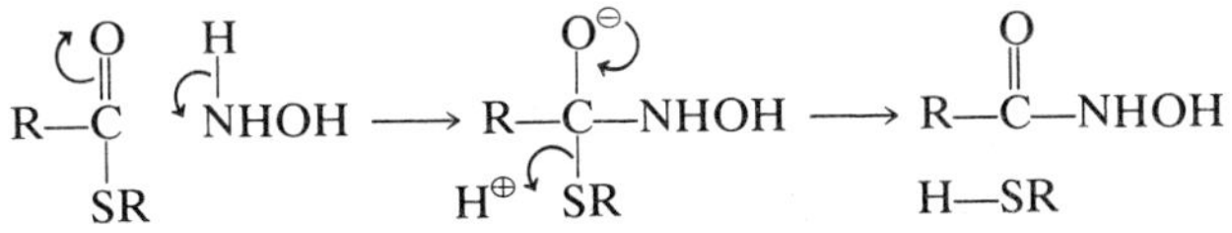

$$R-\overset{\overset{O}{\|}}{\underset{\underset{SR}{|}}{C}} \quad \overset{H}{\underset{NHOH}{|}} \longrightarrow R-\overset{\overset{O^{\ominus}}{|}}{\underset{\underset{H^{\oplus}\,SR}{|}}{C}}-NHOH \longrightarrow R-\overset{\overset{O}{\|}}{C}-NHOH$$

$$H-SR$$

SCHEME 4.12

When we turn to the question of thermodynamic reactivity we move onto firmer ground because this factor is independent of the nature of the intervening steps and is determined solely by the relative stabilities of starting materials and products. We have already seen that this aspect of reactivity is a decisive factor in the controlled working of the metabolic pathways. The expectation that the thioester would be less stable than the equivalent oxygen ester is supported by measurements of the free energy of hydrolysis. Thus an acetyl thioester releases $32\,\text{kJ mol}^{-1}$ and consequently enjoys the status of an energy rich compound, whereas the oxygen ester releases only $21\,\text{kJ mol}^{-1}$ and so is classed as energy-poor. As a result, a process which takes place by cleavage of a thioester rather than an oxygen ester will take place more completely, and therefore will be more effective in driving a metabolic process in the desired direction.

At this point it is worth digressing briefly to consider the apparently conflicting situation in the biosynthesis of proteins where the oxygen ester serves as the reactive derivative of the amino acid building blocks, as shown in Scheme 4.13. The residues $tRNA_x$ represent complex transfer ribonucleic acid molecules each corresponding to a particular amino acid. Their function is to ensure that the amino acids are lined up

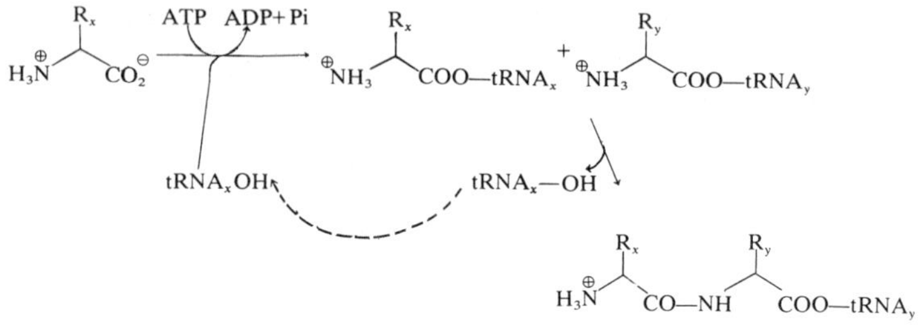

SCHEME 4.13

in the correct sequence for protein formation, but we are not concerned with that aspect of the problem here and so can ignore the details of their structure, apart from noting that the reactive residue which combines with the carboxyl group of the amino acid is an alcoholic hydroxyl group.

The employment of oxygen esters of the amino acids in this vital area of biosynthesis falls into line with the arguments advanced in the previous paragraph as soon as the free energy of hydrolysis is taken into consideration: the typical value of around 35 kJ mol^{-1} is actually higher than that of the thioester of an ordinary carboxylic acid. The increased reactivity of the oxygen ester in the amino acid series can be attributed to the influence of the amino group. The diagrams in Scheme 4.14 illustrate how the inductive effect of this group (which is extensively protonated at pH 7) destabilizes the starting ester on the one hand and stabilizes the products on the other.

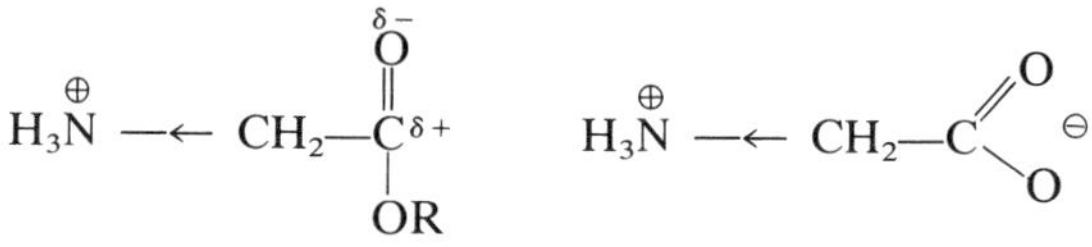

SCHEME 4.14

Thioesters in relation to ATP

At the end of the last chapter we compared the thermodynamic reactivity of the different derivatives of phosphoric acid, and saw how the gradation of reactivity shown by these compounds is exploited in the functioning of the metabolic pathways. At this stage it is useful to undertake a similar survey of the biologically important derivatives of the carboxyl group. To this end the free energies of hydrolysis of the various acyl derivatives are plotted on the left-hand side of Scheme 4.15 with the oxygen ester of a straightforward carboxylic acid included as a basis for comparison. The free energy of hydrolysis of ATP is also plotted on the right to bring out the relationship between this key compound and the different derivatives in the acyl series.

In comparing the relative merits of the thioester and the oxygen ester we have argued that the former would have the advantage of greater thermodynamic reactivity and therefore be more useful in the synthetic sense. In that case how can we account for the widespread use of the thioester in preference to the even more reactive acyl phosphate? From the standpoint of a particular synthetic process taken in isolation, the

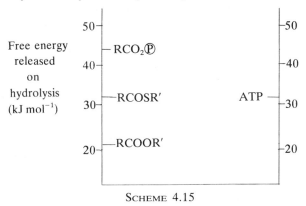

Scheme 4.15

acyl phosphate would indeed be the more effective reactive intermediate, but in the wider context of bioenergetics we have to take into account that frequently the desired intermediate has to be generated from the free carboxylic acid in a reaction driven by the free energy released on hydrolysis of ATP. In this situation the higher reactivity of the acyl phosphate would be disadvantageous because only a relatively small pool of intermediate would be present at any time and therefore the desired synthetic reaction would be hindered in the kinetic sense by a shortage of starting material.

Nevertheless acyl phosphates do play a vital role in metabolism. For example, as we saw in Schemes 4.6 and 4.7, one serves as intermediate in a key process by which a thioester is generated from a carboxylic acid at the expense of ATP. The answer to the apparent conflict between this observation and the arguments advanced above lies in the special character of the enzymes which normally carry out this type of transformation. Almost invariably the intermediate mixed anhydride does not dissociate from the enzyme on which it is formed, but reacts *in situ* with the thiol to generate the desired thioester. This special mode of operation neatly avoids the problem that would arise from having a small pool of the reactive intermediate widely dispersed in solution, but obviously it would not be convenient to have to rely on this stratagem in all processes involving derivatization of the carboxyl group.

So far we have only considered the relative merits of the different acyl derivatives in the sphere of synthesis. We have already seen that such compounds play an equally important role in the degradative reactions of catabolism, where they function in the opposite sense; that is, they are generated as a consequence of an oxidative process and then undergo cleavage with concomitant formation of ATP. Finding the free energy to generate the reactive intermediate is not now a vital consideration, because it is available by virtue of the particular oxidative process. The important consideration is whether the subsequent cleavage of the acyl derivative releases sufficient free energy to drive the formation of ATP. An acyl phosphate qualifies on this basis, as does the thioester of an ordinary acid (just), but the corresponding oxygen ester would not be sufficiently reactive. As we shall see in later chapters both of the former derivatives do serve in this way.

However, taking the overall view, we can now see that it is the thioester group that is ideally qualified to serve as the general factotum in the metabolic chemistry of the acyl group, by virtue of its equivalence with ATP in terms of the free energy of hydrolysis. Thus, a reaction in which the formation and cleavage of these two types of derivative are linked can proceed readily in either direction, and many important aspects of metabolism hinge on this key relationship.

5. Thiamine pyrophosphate and lipoic acid

So far we have concentrated on the way in which the chemical energy stored in ATP is used to drive the thermodynamically unfavourable reactions of metabolism. In the next three chapters we shall be covering the complementary aspect of bioenergetics, that is, how the free energy released in the oxidative reactions of catabolism is harnessed to regenerate ATP.

The major part of this chapter is devoted to the coenzyme thiamine pyrophosphate, and in considering its reactions we shall be mainly concerned with the question of mechanism rather than equilibrium. As a result, we shall digress for a time from the subject of bioenergetics, and the tenor of the discussion will be closer to that of the later chapters dealing with purely catalytic coenzymes such as pyridoxal phosphate. However, it is necessary to cover the reactions of thiamine pyrophosphate at this stage because, as we shall see, it acts as the pivot in one of the key energy-harnessing reactions of metabolism.

Biological reactions of thiamine pyrophosphate

(1) *Degradation of α-keto acids*

Thiamine pyrophosphate is used to catalyse the degradation of α-keto acids in a variety of ways. The range of transformations in the case of pyruvic acid is illustrated below and the reaction schemes show the different fates of this acid when it is produced as an intermediate in the catabolism of glucose. In the diagrams thiamine pyrophosphate is indicated by the standard abbreviation, TPP.

(*a*) *Non-oxidative decarboxylation.* This reaction, shown in Scheme 5.1, is utilized in the breakdown of glucose under anaerobic conditions by yeast. The acetaldehyde is normally reduced to ethanol as we shall see in Chapter 8.

(*b*) *Oxidative decarboxylation.* In the corresponding reaction of aerobic metabolism (Scheme 5.2) the product emerges at the carboxyl

$$CH_3COCO_2H \xrightarrow{\text{TPP}} CH_3CHO + CO_2$$

SCHEME 5.1

level of oxidation (as its coenzyme A ester). The oxidation is carried out at the expense of NAD^+ and therefore ultimately at the expense of molecular oxygen. This reaction and the equivalent reaction on α-ketoglutarate (see Scheme 5.16) represent the key energy-harnessing processes mentioned in the introduction.

$$CH_3COCO_2H \xrightarrow{\text{TPP+other coenzymes}} CH_3COSCoA + CO_2$$
$$\text{CoASH} \quad \text{NAD}^{\oplus} \quad \text{NADH}$$

SCHEME 5.2

(c) *Acetoin formation.* This reaction (Scheme 5.3) is not on the normal pathway of glucose catabolism but is included to illustrate the diversity of reactions catalysed by thiamine pyrophosphate.

$$CH_3COCO_2H + CH_3CHO \xrightarrow{\text{TPP}} CH_3COCHOHCH_3 + CO_2$$

SCHEME 5.3

(2) *Transketolization*

The remarkable diversity of reaction catalysed by thiamine pyrophosphate is further illustrated by the next reaction which plays an important part in carbohydrate anabolism. In the overall process a C_2 unit (shown in heavy type in Scheme 5.4) is transferred from one molecule to another. The groups R^1 and R^2 represent different carbohydrate residues and several examples of this reaction can be found on the pathways of carbohydrate biosynthesis. Note that the process can operate usefully in either direction.

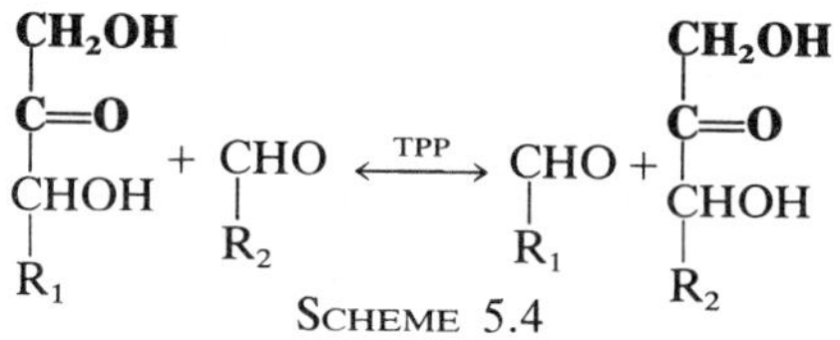

$$\begin{array}{ccc} \textbf{CH}_2\textbf{OH} & & \textbf{CH}_2\textbf{OH} \\ | & & | \\ \textbf{C}{=}\textbf{O} & \text{CHO} & \text{CHO} & \textbf{C}{=}\textbf{O} \\ | & + \; | \; \xleftarrow{\text{TPP}} \; | \; + & | \\ \text{CHOH} & R_2 & R_1 & \text{CHOH} \\ | & & | \\ R_1 & & R_2 \end{array}$$

SCHEME 5.4

Mechanism of action

The mechanism of action of thiamine pyrophosphate is a fascinating topic, if only because several of the reactions it catalyses have no close analogy in organic chemistry; moreover at first sight it would appear that the only connection between the four types of reaction is the fact that they are all catalysed by the one coenzyme. However, the transformations do have a common rationale in terms of mechanism, and the biochemistry of this coenzyme nicely illustrates the advantage of the mechanistic approach.

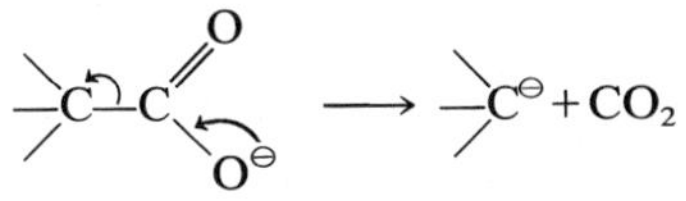

$$\text{Scheme 5.5}$$

Before considering the question of how the coenzyme produces its catalytic effect, it is useful to consider the reactions themselves from the mechanistic point of view, starting with the simplest, the decarboxylation of pyruvic acid to give acetaldehyde. One possible mechanism involves the formation of a carbanion, as in Scheme 5.5, followed by protonation. In the case of the enzymic decarboxylation of pyruvic acid this mechanism would lead to the intermediate **carbanion [30]** as shown in Scheme 5.6. Significantly the same intermediate or its equivalent [31] could be invoked in each of the remaining reactions, and this point is illustrated for acetoin formation in Scheme 5.7.

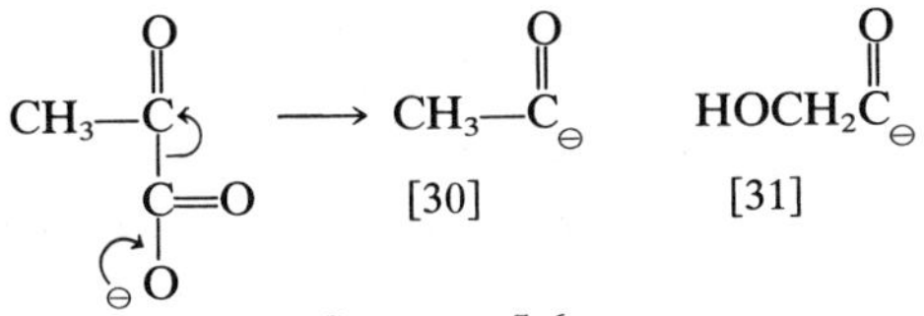

$$\text{Scheme 5.6}$$

While this simple view nicely correlates the reactions into a common mechanistic scheme, it fails to take into account the unstable character of the proposed intermediate. Carbanions of this type are not observed as intermediates in organic chemistry, and it is significant that the organic chemist has to employ an indirect approach, such as that illustrated in Scheme 5.8, when he wishes to generate a species equivalent to this carbanion. Many readers will no doubt be familiar with this particular stratagem: the carbonyl group is temporarily converted to a dithian derivative [32], and the carbanion [33] can then be generated in which the negative charge on the relevant carbon is stabilized by interaction with the neighbouring sulphur atoms. The carbonyl group is regenerated on completion of the desired reaction, in this example a deuteration.

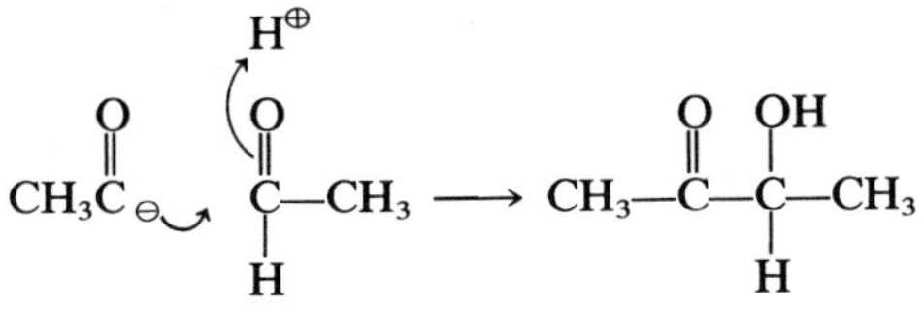

$$\text{Scheme 5.7}$$

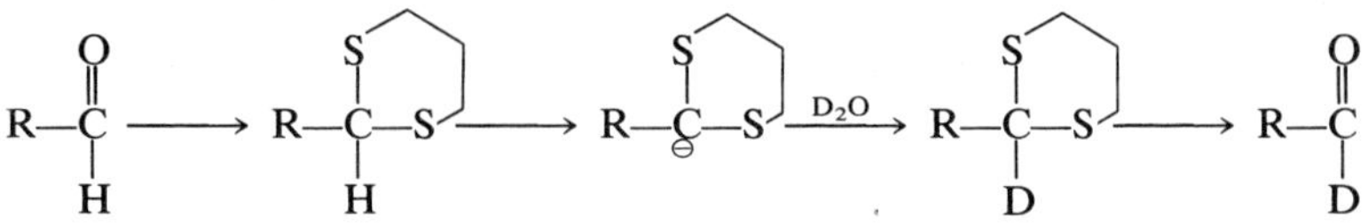

SCHEME 5.8

It was long suspected that thiamine pyrophosphate might exert its catalytic effect in the biological reactions in an equivalent way; that is, that by suitably modifying the reactivity of the carbonyl group it might facilitate the generation of a carbanion on the relevant carbon. The question is how this might be achieved, and this problem exercised the imagination of chemists for many years before the correct answer was discovered.

The problem is that, unlike ATP and coenzyme A, this coenzyme emerges from each of its reactions without apparent change, so there is no obvious clue as to the site of catalytic activity from any observable change in structure. The structure of the coenzyme, [34] is remarkably inscrutable in that there is no residue which stands out as the probable site of activity. Nevertheless, many plausible proposals were put forward by early workers to account for the mechanism of action. For example mechanisms were proposed based on catalysis by one or other of the two functional groups marked by an arrow in the structure, and other mechanisms invoked cleavage of the thiazolidine ring to provide a suitable catalytic site. In the event, none of these early proposals proved to be correct and it was found that the site of catalytic activity resided in the intact thiazolidine ring. Accordingly, the abbreviated structure [35] will be used from now on.

The vital clue which led to the solution of the mystery came from an n.m.r. experiment in which it was discovered that the hydrogen of the thiazolidine ring is readily replaced by deuterium in D_2O solution at pH 7. The most plausible mechanism for this exchange is shown in Scheme 5.9.

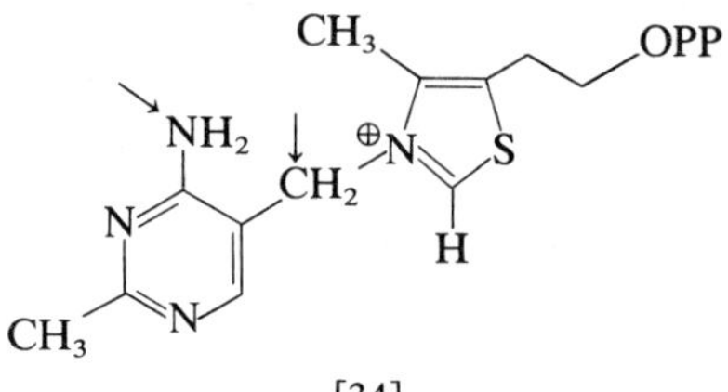

[34] 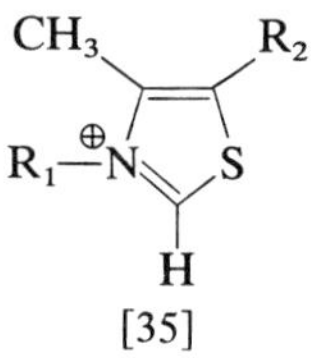   [35]

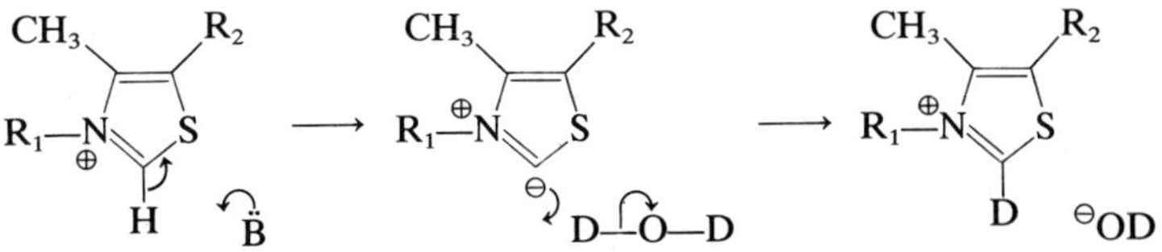

SCHEME 5.9

This explanation assumes that the carbanion [36] should be reasonably stable and with the benefit of hindsight one can recognize two influences to account for this unexpected phenomenon: firstly, interaction of the carbanion with the neighbouring sulphur atom as in the case of the dithian anion, [33], and secondly the favourable inductive effect of the adjacent positively charged nitrogen atom. The exchange reactions shown in Scheme 5.10 presumably go via carbanion intermediates and therefore provide a precedent for the latter effect.

Thus the organic chemist will recognize that the carbanion [36] is a member of the extensive family of ylides, in which a carbanion is stabilized by the presense of an adjacent nitrogen, sulphur, or phosphorus atom. Nevertheless, in this case the degree of stability is exceptional and it is not surprising that early workers in this field failed to anticipate this property of the thiazolidine ring.

With the help of this clue the problem of accounting for the catalytic effect of the coenzyme becomes relatively straightforward, and the reaction sequence in Scheme 5.11 shows a mechanism for the decarboxylation of pyruvic acid. In the first step a nucleophilic addition to the carbon of the carbonyl group alters its reactivity in such a way that the carbanion generated at that position in the key decarboxylation step is stabilized by delocalization, as shown below in structure [37]. The thiazolidine ring acts as a very effective electron sink and so subsequent mechanistic schemes will show this intermediate as the equivalent

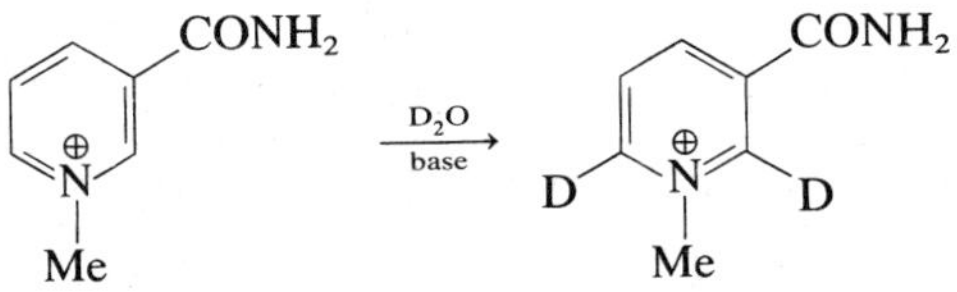

SCHEME 5.10

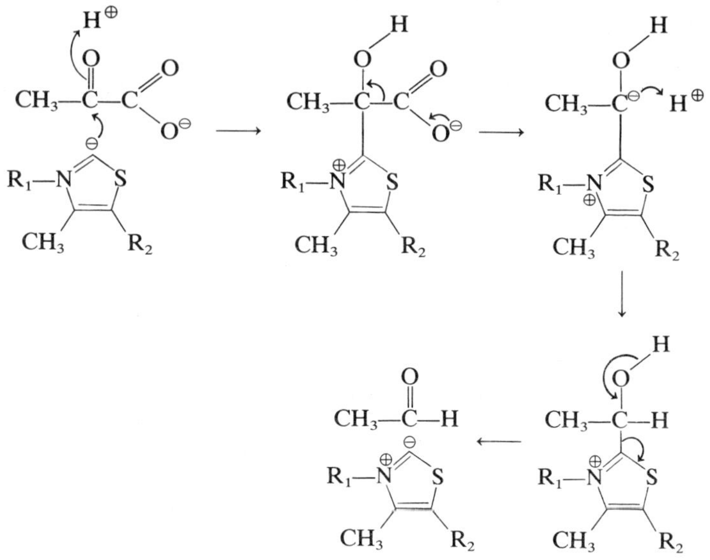

SCHEME 5.11

enamine form [38]. Indeed, this intermediate in its protonated form [39] has been isolated from some enzyme-mediated reactions.

In the case of acetoin formation this same intermediate is formed in an identical way but subsequently undergoes nucleophilic attack on a molecule of acetaldehyde as shown in Scheme 5.12.

It is interesting to note that there is a good analogy for this process in the catalysis of the familiar benzoin condensation by cyanide ion. In each case the catalyst meets three essential requirements: in the first step it acts as a good nucleophile in adding to the carbonyl group; secondly, having added it can serve as an electron sink to stabilize an anionic intermediate; and thirdly, it can act as a good leaving group to regenerate the carbonyl group in the final step.

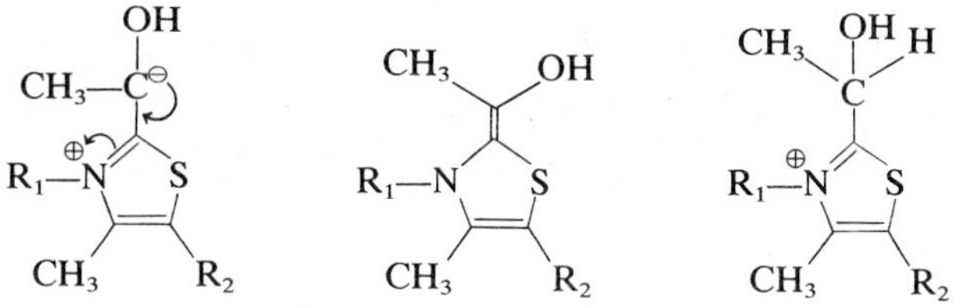

[37]   [38]   [39]

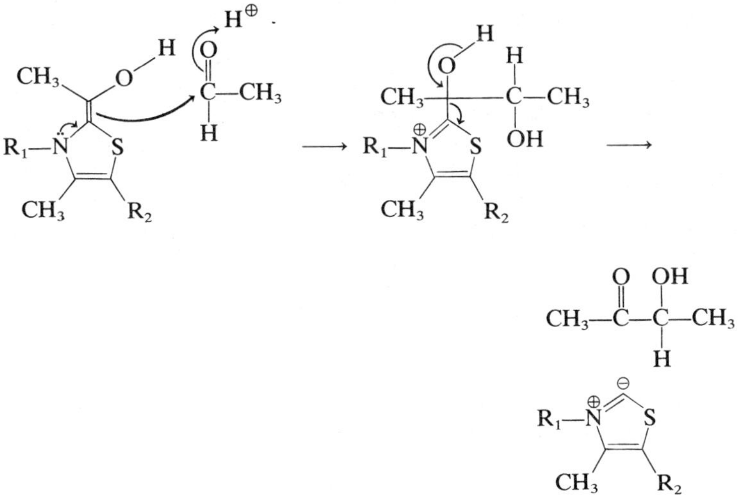

SCHEME 5.12

The mechanistic Scheme 5.13 for the first steps of transketolization has the same underlying rationale though there is a difference in the structure of the intermediate, [40] as opposed to [38], corresponding to the nature of the group undergoing transfer. The rest of the process is merely the reverse of the steps shown, but with a different aldehyde.

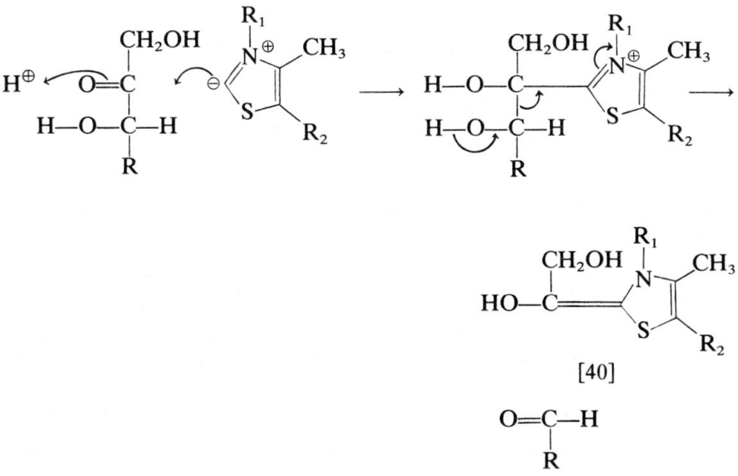

SCHEME 5.13

Oxidative decarboxylation of α-keto acids: mechanism and bioenergetics

With the oxidative decarboxylation of α-keto acids we come to the *pièce de resistance* in the repertoire of reactions catalysed by thiamine pyrophosphate. The reaction is extraordinarily complex in that it involves a cast of no less than five coenzymes, and takes place on a multi-enzyme apparatus of exceptional complexity.

Two of the coenzymes, thiamine pyrophosphate and coenzyme A, are already familiar. The remaining three, NADH, FAD, and lipoic acid have not been covered in detail yet. However, only the latter contributes directly to the process of decarboxylation and so needs to be discussed in detail at this stage. The NADH and FAD fulfil a peripheral role which will be explained in outline only in this chapter.

The structure of lipoic acid [41] shows how the coenzyme is covalently bound to a lysine unit of the protein chain of the enzyme via an amide derivative of its carboxyl group. As usual the catalytically active residue

Lipoic acid residue   Lysine residue

[41]

is shown in heavy type. It is proposed that the initial steps of the oxidative decarboxylation are the same as those of non-oxidative decarboxylation leading to the key intermediate [38]. At this point the oxidative pathway diverges to follow the steps shown in Scheme 5.14. The proposed mechanism of oxidation by lipoic acid, [38] → [42], is purely speculative. In [42] the key carbon is at the carboxyl level of oxidation so that subsequent release of the thiamine pyrophosphate results in the generation of an enzyme-bound thioester [43]. Finally the acyl group is removed from the enzyme by transfer to the thiol group of coenzyme A in the usual way. The process of oxidative decarboxylation is now complete but the lipoic acid is left in its reduced form [44]. It is reoxidized to the disulphide by NAD$^+$ with the intermediacy of a second coenzyme, FAD, as in Scheme 5.15. The NADH is reoxidized elsewhere and the complete system is ready to operate on the next molecule of ketoacid.

While these reactions make a fascinating study on the basis of mechanism alone, the cunning design and resourcefulness of the system can be fully appreciated only when the efficiency of the overall process in terms of energy conservation is taken into account. This aspect of the

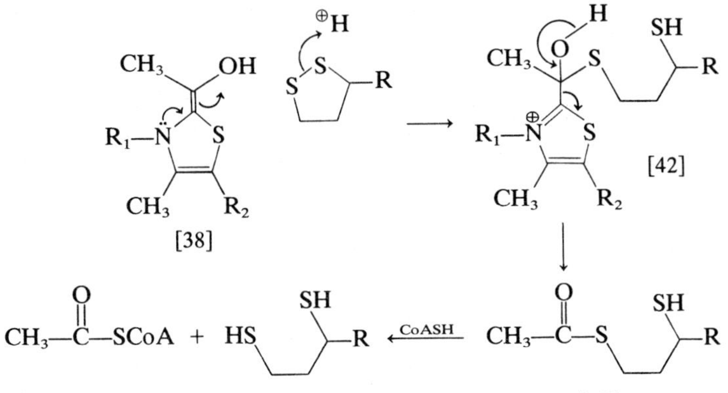

SCHEME 5.14

problem will be illustrated by considering the role of an equivalent reaction, the oxidative decarboxylation of α-ketoglutarate [45] to give the coenzyme A ester of succinic acid. This is one of the steps of the citric acid cycle which will be discussed in full in Chapter 8. At this stage it is sufficient to know that, in the next step of the sequence, the thioester is hydrolysed to yield succinic acid with concomitant formation of an ATP equivalent in the form of the nucleoside triphosphate, guanosine triphosphate (GTP). The sequence is illustrated in Scheme 5.16 and the diagram as a whole is intended to show how the reactions fit into the wider plan of metabolism. Thus the molecule of coenzyme A after liberation by hydrolysis is free to return to the decarboxylation system, so that, in effect, its contribution is to act as a carrier of the acyl derivative in the form of a thioester from one enzyme to another. The other coenzyme we have to account for is the NAD^+ which was reduced in the reoxidation of dihydrolipoic acid (Scheme 5.15). This will normally be regenerated by oxidation in the electron transport system as shown. The net result of all these steps is that the α-ketoglutaric acid has been oxidized to succinic acid, ultimately at the expense of the oxygen supplied to the electron transport system, and in addition several molecules of ATP have been generated.

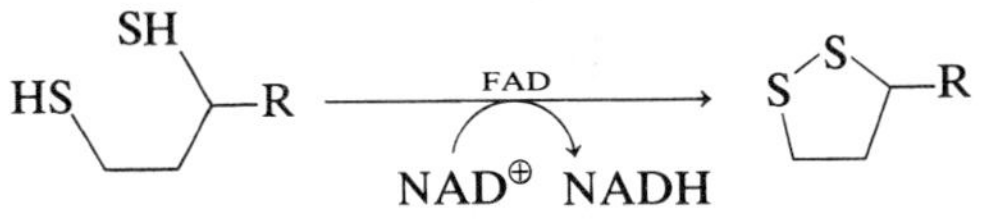

SCHEME 5.15

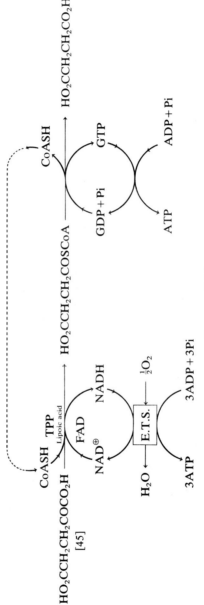

SCHEME 5.16

In considering the process from the point of view of bioenergetics we are interested in the formation of ATP and it is apparent from Scheme 5.16 that, in all, four molecules are generated for each molecule of keto acid oxidized: three in the electron transport system and a fourth as a consequence of thioester hydrolysis. Obviously the more ATP that can be generated the greater the efficiency of the overall process and it is this factor which accounts for the otherwise puzzling complexity of the oxidative decarboxylation process.

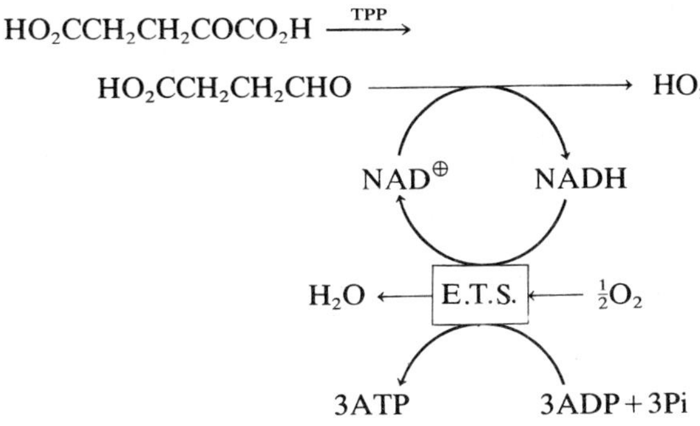

$$HO_2CCH_2CH_2COCO_2H \xrightarrow{\text{TPP}}$$

$$HO_2CCH_2CH_2CHO \longrightarrow HO_2CCH_2CH_2CO_2H$$

NAD$^{\oplus}$ NADH

H$_2$O ← E.T.S. ← $\frac{1}{2}$O$_2$

3ATP   3ADP + 3Pi

SCHEME 5.17

In order to illustrate this point a hypothetical sequence of reactions is proposed in Scheme 5.17, by which the overall oxidative decarboxylation would be achieved in just two enzyme-mediated reactions, each of a standard type, with the assistance of only two coenzymes. However, although this hypothetical scheme for oxidative decarboxylation has the advantage of simplicity, it also has the very serious disadvantage, that only three molecules of ATP would be generated per cycle instead of four. Thus the extraordinary complexity of the system which has actually evolved to carry out the process is not the unfortunate outcome of a wrong turn at an early stage in the evolution of the metabolic pathways; in fact it results in a significantly higher efficiency of energy conservation and the first living system to develop this complex process would have reaped a significant advantage in the evolutionary struggle.

6. The coenzymes of hydrogen transfer: the nicotinamides and the flavins

In this chapter we shall be covering reactions in which a substrate is oxidized (or reduced) by transfer of two hydrogens to (or from) a coenzyme. This is by far the most important class of redox reaction that takes place on the metabolic pathways and we have already met a key example in the last chapter in the reoxidation of dihydrolipoic acid (Scheme 5.15) which takes place by removal of two hydrogens with the coenzyme NAD^+ acting as acceptor.

We have already seen in outline how reactions of this type contribute to the energy requirements of the cell by providing NADH as fuel for the electron transport system. However, detailed consideration of that aspect of the subject can wait until the next chapter and for the moment we will focus our attention on the question of mechanism in the various types of hydrogen transfer process.

Most of the reactions under consideration are capable of operating in either direction. Consequently we shall be concerned not only with the oxidative type of process characteristic of catabolism pathways but also with processes of the opposite type (usually synthetic) in which the substrate undergoes reduction by accepting two hydrogens from the reduced form of coenzyme. In all four coenzymes serve in this way and they share the general pattern of operation which is illustrated in Scheme 6.1 where the coenzyme is shown operating in two separate reactions. Firstly, it acts as an oxidizing agent by accepting two hydrogens from a substrate, AH_2; then the coenzyme, in its reduced form, donates two hydrogens to reduce a second substrate B. The coenzyme is now ready to repeat the cycle and it can be seen to act, in effect, as a carrier of hydrogen between the two substrates AH_2 and B. The mode of operation of NAD^+ in glucose catabolism fits into this general pattern, with B representing the initial oxidizing agent of the electron transport system and AH_2 the catabolic intermediate undergoing oxidation. However, reaction cycles of this type also service the synthetic pathways of anabolism by supplying reduced coenzymes to carry out the requisite

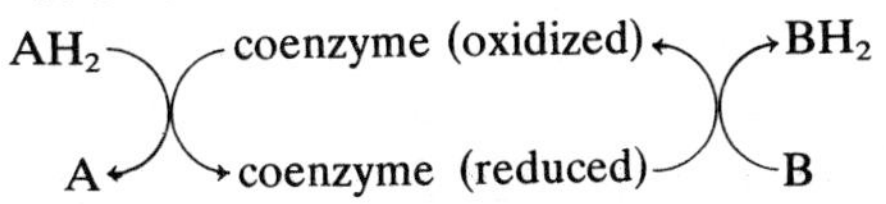

$$AH_2 \quad \text{coenzyme (oxidized)} \quad BH_2$$
$$A \quad \text{coenzyme (reduced)} \quad B$$

SCHEME 6.1

reduction steps. In this situation B would represent the anabolic intermediate undergoing reduction and AH_2 the immediate source of reducing power.

The coenzymes which operate in this way are classified as nicotinamide or flavin according to the structure of the operative part
and there are two representatives of each type. Although they show
important differences in their mode of operation the two categories of
coenzyme will be covered together in this chapter, partly because they
are so closely related in function, and, more importantly, because it is
helpful to compare them from the mechanistic point of view.

The nicotinamide coenzymes

Structure

The full structure of NAD (nicotinamide adenine dinucleotide) is
shown [46] with the site of reaction emphasized by heavy type in the
usual way. In passing it is interesting to note that a major part of the
non-operative residue corresponds to a molecule of ADP, and so this

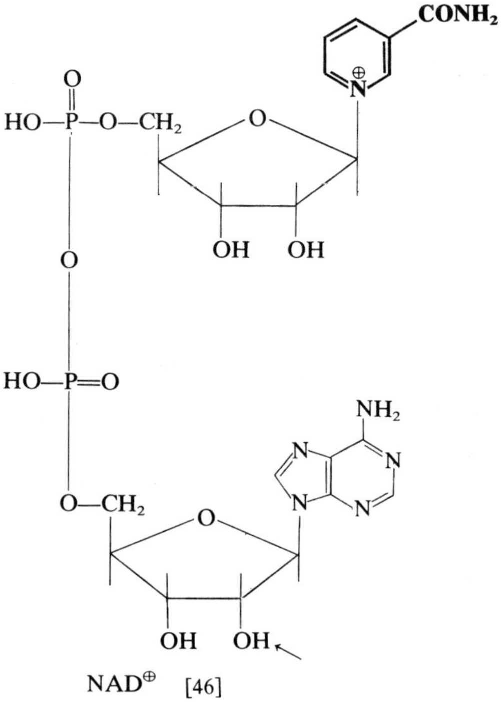

$$NAD^\oplus \quad [46]$$

key nucleotide structure makes its presence felt in yet another coenzyme, albeit in an indirect way by contributing to enzyme recognition and binding.

In the subsequent discussion the partial structure [47] will be used. When the coenzyme accepts two hydrogens in a biological reaction this residue is converted as shown in Scheme 6.2 to a 1,4-dihydropyridine derivative, [48], which thus represents the partial structure of NADH. Note that, since the nitrogen is only weakly basic, the predominant species at neutral pH is the unprotonated form of the dihydropyridine as shown.

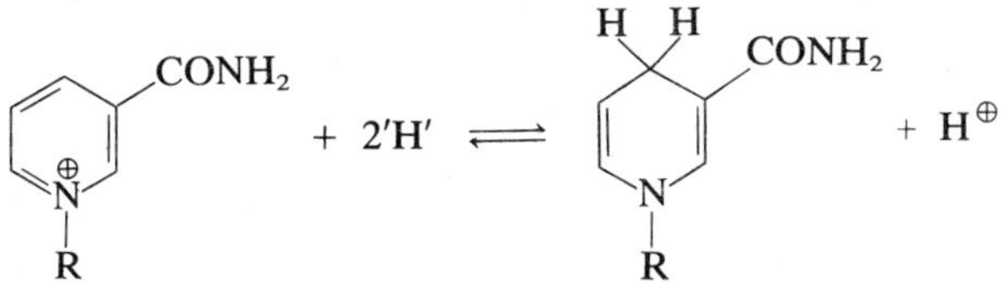

SCHEME 6.2

The second nicotinamide coenzyme couple, $NADP^+/NADPH$, has the same working part as the first and, since it functions in an identical manner, the one partial structure will serve for both. The difference in structure between the two coenzymes lies at the hydroxyl group marked by an arrow in [46]. In $NADP^+$, this group is esterified to form a monophosphate ester and it is this 'extra' phosphate group which is specified in the full name of the coenzyme (nicotinamide adenine dinucleotide phosphate), and in the initials derived from it.

Slight though it may seem, this difference in the structure of the 'handle' is sufficient to ensure that, with very few exceptions, a particular enzyme will work with one coenzyme couple or the other but not with both. As a result the two pools of coenzyme are virtually independent of each other, and it is interesting to note that the synthetic pathways of anabolism employ the couple $NADP^+/NADPH$ acting in the reducing sense, whereas the oxidative reactions of catabolism are the preserve of the couple $NAD^+/NADH$. Although not absolutely clear-cut, this division of function helps to keep separate these two conflicting aspects of metabolism, and thus contributes to the ordered working of the metabolic machine.

Metabolic reactions

Taken together, the two nicotinamide coenzymes play a part in most aspects of metabolism and the total number of enzymes with which they serve as cofactor runs into three figures. Fortunately the range of reactions is not so extensive because a particular type of transformation may be catalysed by many different enzymes each operating on its own substrate or limited range of substrates. In addition, the two coenzymes carry out the same range of reactions even though they function in the different spheres of catabolism and anabolism. Nevertheless the list of reactions shown in Scheme 6.3 is impressive even though only the straightforward types of reaction effected by these coenzymes are shown. Other more specialized applications in which a nicotinamide coenzyme acts in cooperation with one of the flavin coenzymes will be discussed later.

The first reaction is a standard interconversion of an alcohol with the corresponding aldehyde or ketone. The inherent equilibrium usually favours the alcohol; however, it is pH-dependent and can be moved in favour of the aldehyde by increasing the pH. In the context of a metabolic pathway the process can operate usefully in either direction.

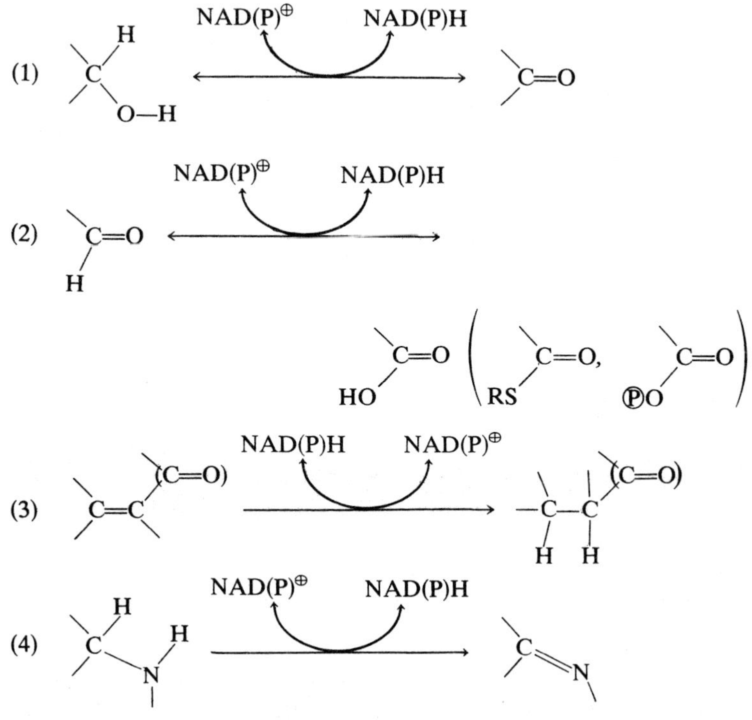

SCHEME 6.3

In the second reaction an aldehyde is oxidized to an acyl derivative and the product may be released as the free acid or as one of the two standard derivatives shown, depending on the enzyme involved. The interconversion of an aldehyde with a high-energy acyl derivative (i.e. a thiol ester or an acyl phosphate) will operate usefully in either direction depending on the metabolic pathway. However, in the oxidation of an aldehyde to the much more stable free carboxylic acid the reaction will not operate usefully in the reverse direction because the equilibrium lies so completely on the side of the acid. Therefore a free carboxylic acid is always activated by conversion to one of the two standard high-energy derivatives before reduction to the aldehyde on the appropriate enzyme.

The third reaction shows the coenzyme reducing a carbon–carbon double bond, which may be either an isolated double bond or one conjugated with a carbonyl group. The process normally operates in the direction shown and many important anabolic pathways involve one or more reactions of this type. In the fourth reaction, the coenzyme is shown interconverting an imine and an amine. Unlike the others, this reaction is not on the main stream of metabolism, but is included for its interest from the chemical point of view.

This list demonstrates the extraordinary versatility of the nicotinamide coenzymes. Though many of the reactions can be carried out conveniently and in high yield in the laboratory, others, such as the oxidation of a primary alcohol to an aldehyde (avoiding carboxylic acid formation), or the oxidation of an amine to an imine, are less easy to duplicate. Moreover, there is no one reagent available to the organic chemist which can match the all-round ability of the coenzyme to carry out every one of the reactions listed.

Mechanism of action

Of the reactions listed in Scheme 6.3 the first has been studied most thoroughly from the mechanistic point of view, and therefore provides the best basis for the discussion in this section. The process is catalysed by a family of enzymes called the alcohol dehydrogenases. Enzymes of this type can be isolated from a variety of sources (e.g. yeast or liver) and they vary according to the structure of the alcohol (or range of alcohols) that they will accept as substrate.

In formal terms the reaction involves the transfer of two hydrogens between the substrate and coenzyme. The fate of these hydrogens during the course of the reaction has been investigated by isotopic labelling experiments. The example shown in Scheme 6.4 is typical and from it one can draw two conclusions. Firstly, that of the two hydrogens undergoing reaction one is transferred between the carbon of the substrate and the carbon of the coenzyme, and, secondly, that in the process

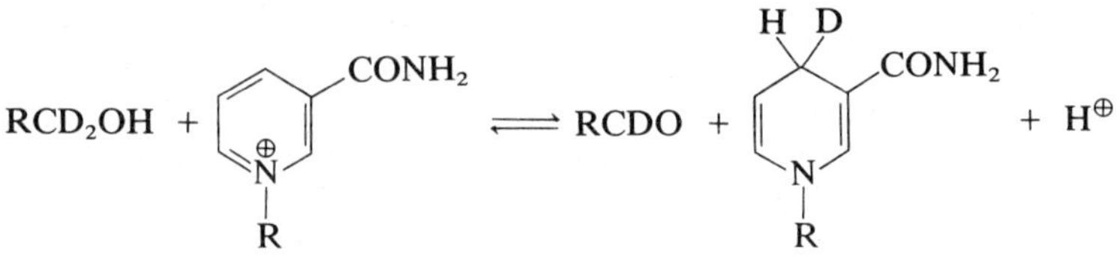

SCHEME 6.4

this hydrogen does not suffer exchange with protons of the medium. The course of the reaction has been probed more deeply using substrates labelled stereospecifically with hydrogen isotopes as illustrated in Scheme 6.5. In this way it has been established that the reaction is stereospecific with respect to the methylene groups of both substrate and reduced coenzyme, so that in each case only one of the two hydrogens is subject to transfer, i.e. the one labelled with deuterium in Scheme 6.5. The second hydrogen which undergoes transfer is, of course, readily exchangeable with the medium, so its fate is not amenable to study by this type of experiment.

By establishing the direction of hydrogen transfer these results define the gross features of the mechanism but they give no information on the nature of the two hydrogen species which undergo transfer. At this stage it seems reasonable to assume that the hydrogen which equilibrates with the medium is transferred as a proton, but, for the hydrogen which migrates from carbon to carbon, one can consider four fundamentally different mechanisms involving transfer as a hydride ion, as a proton, as a hydrogen atom in a radical reaction, or as part of a pericyclic process.

Detailed schemes are given to illustrate two of these possible mechanisms. That in Scheme 6.6 shows how a hydride transfer may take place from coenzyme to the carbonyl group. Scheme 6.7 shows an equivalent process in which the transfer takes place by migration of a hydrogen atom followed by a single electron. Of course, in the latter scheme the timing of these two transfers is yet another variable to be considered, for the reaction could take place equally well with transfer of the electron preceding that of the hydrogen atom. Further detailed schemes could be advanced on the basis of the proton transfer and pericyclic mechanisms

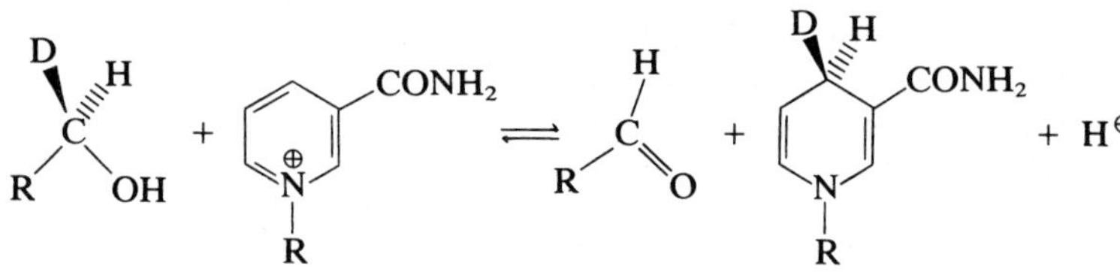

SCHEME 6.5

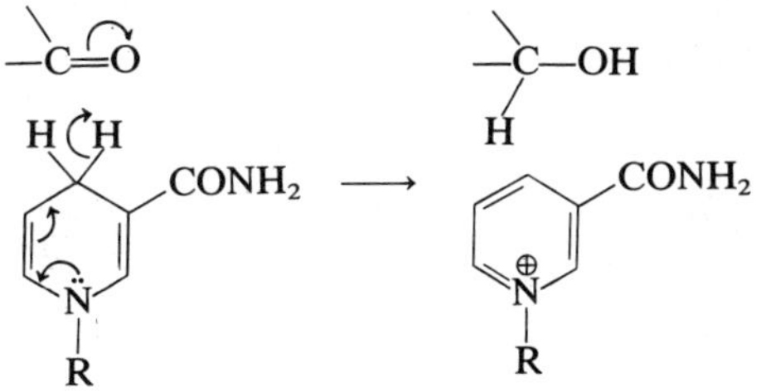

SCHEME 6.6

but the two given are sufficient to indicate the essence of the problem to be solved. At present there is no direct evidence from studies on the enzymic reaction itself to indicate which mechanism is in operation, and at this stage one has to rely on intuition guided by knowledge of the general chemical behaviour of the species undergoing reaction.

On this basis, the hydride mechanism shown in Scheme 6.6 is probably the favoured candidate. Thus the process has analogies in many of the standard chemical methods of reduction of aldehydes and ketones by hydride donors and two examples are illustrated in Scheme 6.8. The borohydride reduction [49] needs no comment but in connection with the Oppenauer oxidation [50] it is interesting to note that there is not only a carbonyl group acting as a hydride acceptor but also an alkoxide acting as a hydride donor, as would be required for the enzymic reaction operating in the direction opposite to that shown in Scheme 6.6.

As far as the coenzyme is concerned, the hydride mechanism accords well with the general chemistry of simple pyridine analogues. Thus N-alkylated pyridinium compounds such as [51] react readily and reversibly at the 2- and 4-positions of the ring with a variety of nucleophiles, and an example is shown for the 4-position in Scheme 6.9. However, in the usual examples of this type of reaction the nucleophile is of a

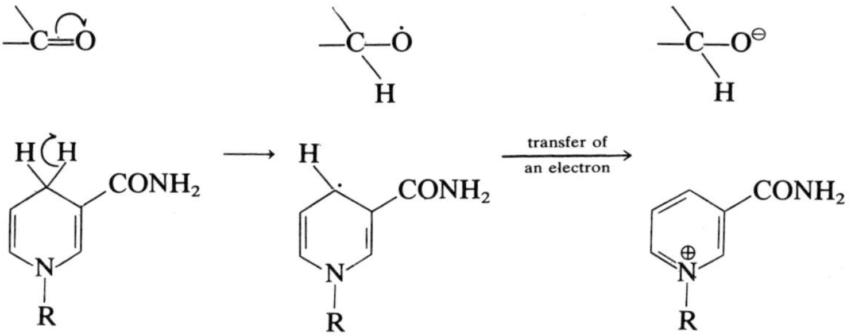

SCHEME 6.7

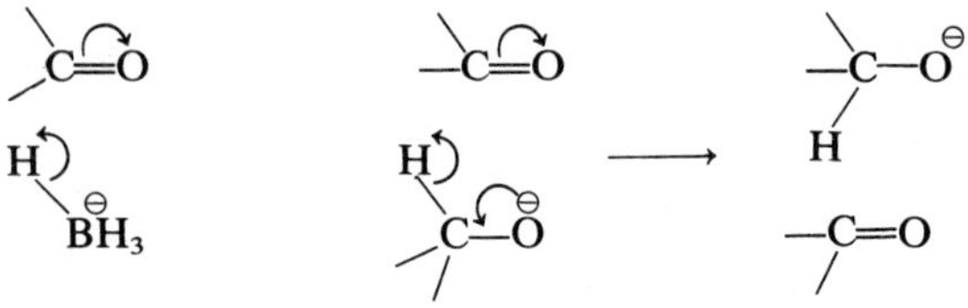

[49]   [50]

SCHEME 6.8

standard type such as hydroxide or cyanide ion and so, spurred by an interest in the mechanism of action of the coenzyme, many investigators have searched for a more closely analogous model reaction in which a dihydropyridine donates a hydride ion to reduce the carbonyl group of a ketone or aldehyde.

In the early work in this field it was found that simple dihydro-pyridines are extremely unstable (as indeed is the coenzyme in solution) and, though they readily act as reducing agents for a wide variety of powerful oxidizing agents (mainly quinonoid compounds), they were found to be disappointingly ineffective in attempted reductions of a simple carbonyl group. Eventually Westheimer discovered the fairly close model reaction shown in Scheme 6.10 in which a more powerfully electrophilic thiocarbonyl group is reduced by hydrogen transfer from a dihydropyridine derivative. In a full investigation of the mechanism of this reaction it has been proved that in the rate-determining step hydrogen is transferred from the dihydropyridine to the thiocarbonyl group, and the inability of radical traps to influence the rate provided evidence against a radical mechanism and thus in favour of the hydride transfer process shown.

This reaction provides a reasonably close analogy for the enzymic reaction but one which bears an even closer resemblance has been

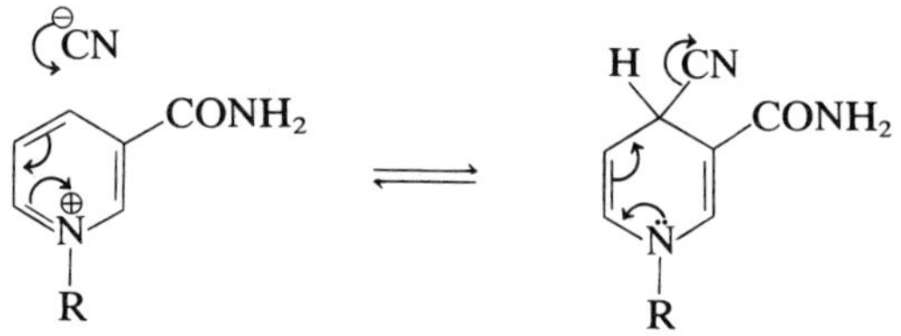

[51]

SCHEME 6.9

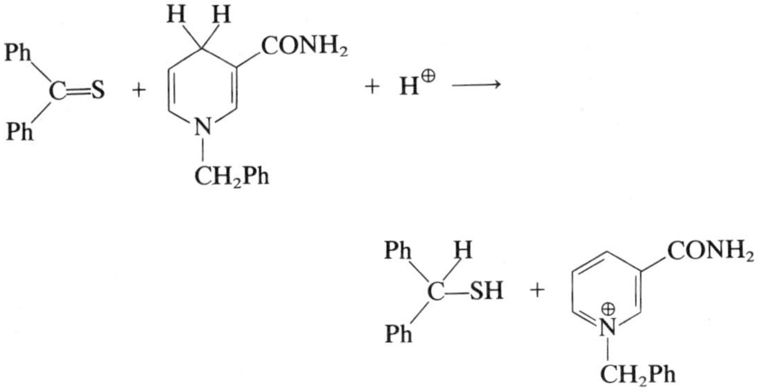

SCHEME 6.10

reported more recently. This reaction is shown in Scheme 6.11 and in it an ordinary carbonyl group is reduced by a dihydropyridine. The secret of the success of this model probably lies in the enhancement of the reactivity of the carbonyl group by coordination with zinc. This ploy is particularly interesting because many alcohol dehydrogenase enzymes contain this metal, which is, moreover, essential for enzymic activity, and it has long been thought possible that the zinc might play its part in the enzymic reaction by coordinating with the carbonyl group in a similar way.

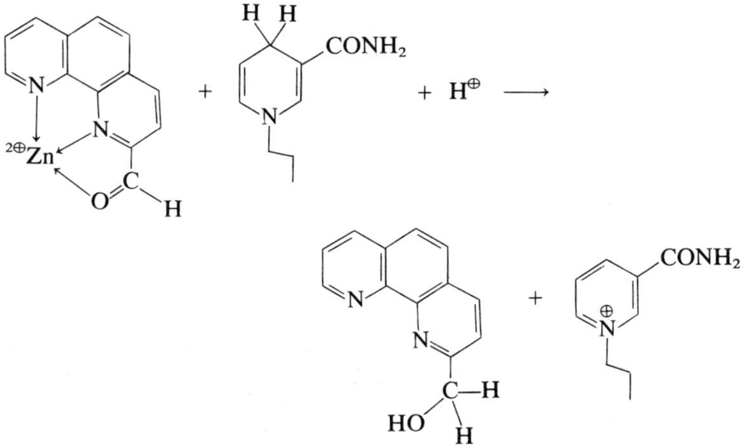

SCHEME 6.11

With the success of this very close model reaction one can feel more confident that the enzymic reaction also proceeds by a direct transfer of a hydride species between the coenzyme and carbonyl group via a transition state such as that shown in Scheme 6.12. Note that the proposed relative orientation of the two reactants is based on the results of the stereospecific labelling experiments described earlier. However, it must be borne in mind that the experimental support for the electronic mechanism comes entirely from the results of model experiments and there is an urgent need for definitive experiments carried out directly on the enzymic reaction.

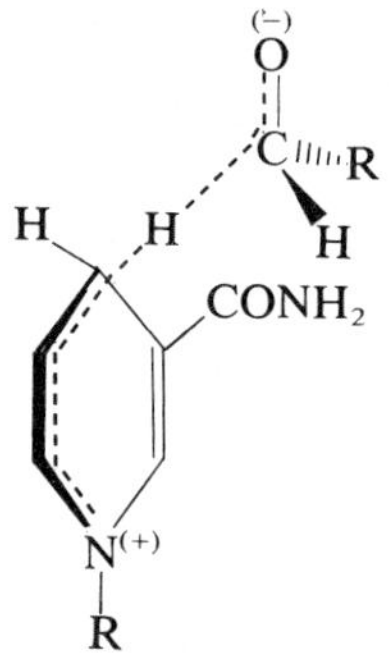

SCHEME 6.12

The other reactions listed in Scheme 6.3 will not be covered in detail because they have not been studied to the same extent and it would involve repetition to survey what little work has been done. Nevertheless they remain a challenging problem for future workers, for whatever mechanism may emerge from the study of the alcohol dehydrogenase enzymes, there is no guarantee that it will apply generally and the coenzyme may work in an entirely different way in other reactions.

The flavin coenzymes

Structure

The oxidized form of one of the flavin coenzymes, FAD (flavin adenine dinucleotide) [52] is shown with the active part (the flavin residue) in heavy type. The coenzyme will be denoted henceforth by the partial structure [53]. The normal reduced form of the coenzyme is the dihydro derivative [54], usually denoted by the initials, FADH$_2$.

The second flavin coenzyme FMN (flavin mononucleotide) has the same operative part but the 'handle' is markedly different: a hydrogen replaces the adenosyl monophosphate residue on the right of the dotted

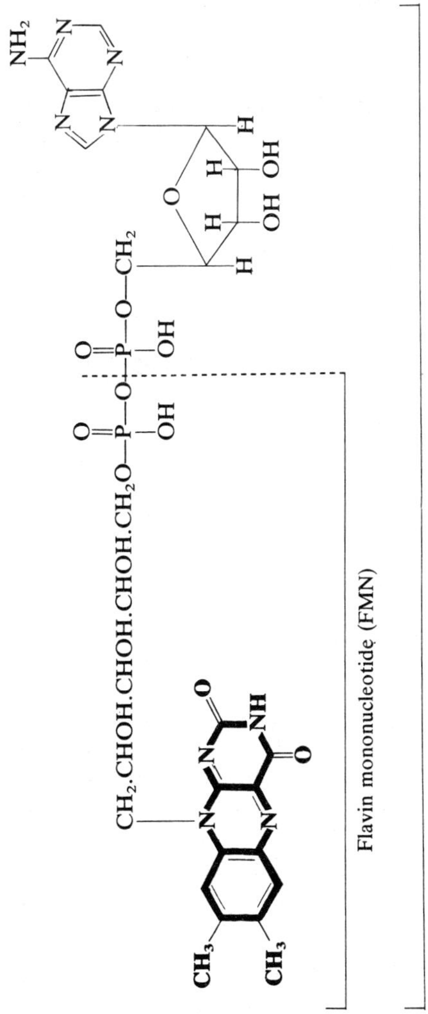

NH_2

$CH_2.CHOH.CHOH.CHOH.CH_2O$

Flavin mononucleotide (FMN)

Flavin adenine dinucleotide (FAD)

[52]

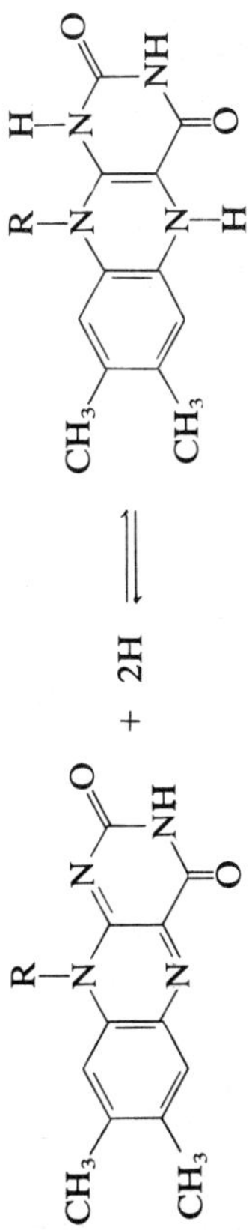

$+ 2H$

[53]

[54]

CH_3

CH_3

line in [52]. The two flavin coenzymes show no apparent division of role in metabolism such as that observed in the case of the nicotinamides.

Metabolic reactions

Although they fulfill the same function in metabolism as the nicotinamides (that of hydrogen transfer from one substrate to another), the flavins operate in a significantly different way. Usually the flavin is very tightly bound to the enzyme with which it operates so that it can almost be regarded as a prosthetic group rather than a coenzyme. (A prosthetic group is a catalytic residue which is not a part of the protein framework of the enzyme but is tightly bound to it and is in effect an integral part of the total enzyme structure. Usually a flavin coenzyme can be dissociated from its protein by treatment with strong acid and so is not a prosthetic group in the strict sense of the definition.) In recognition of this fact the enzyme-coenzyme complex is usually viewed as an entity and called a flavoprotein. The effect of this tight binding on the pattern of operation is illustrated in Scheme 6.13 which shows how, in a normal cycle of reactions, the flavin stays with its enzyme, and the two substrates AH_2 and B travel to it in succession, perhaps reacting at the same catalytic site with the assistance of the same catalytic groups of the enzyme. On the other hand, a nicotinamide coenzyme, in a typical cycle, travels back and forth between two separate enzymes. Thus the catalytic activity of an enzyme employing a nicotinamide cofactor can be adequately discribed in terms of one substrate and one reaction; in the case of a flavoprotein it is necessary to specify two substrates and two reactions.

Scheme 6.14 shows a list of typical hydrogen transfers that can be carried out by flavoproteins. The usual hydrogen acceptor for each type of donor is given on the right: thus in the first two reactions the flavoprotein is reoxidized by direct transfer of hydrogen to molecular

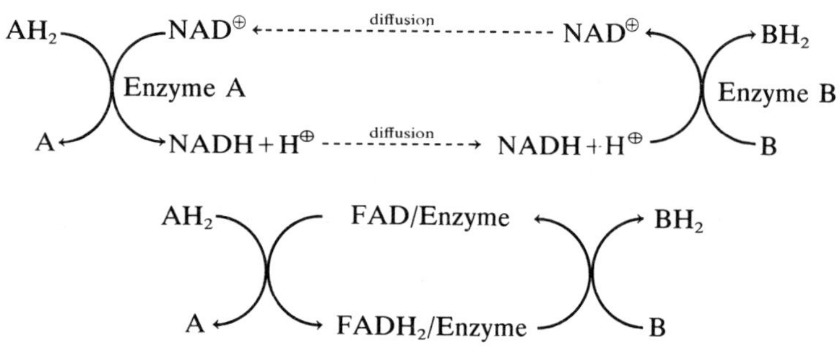

SCHEME 6.13

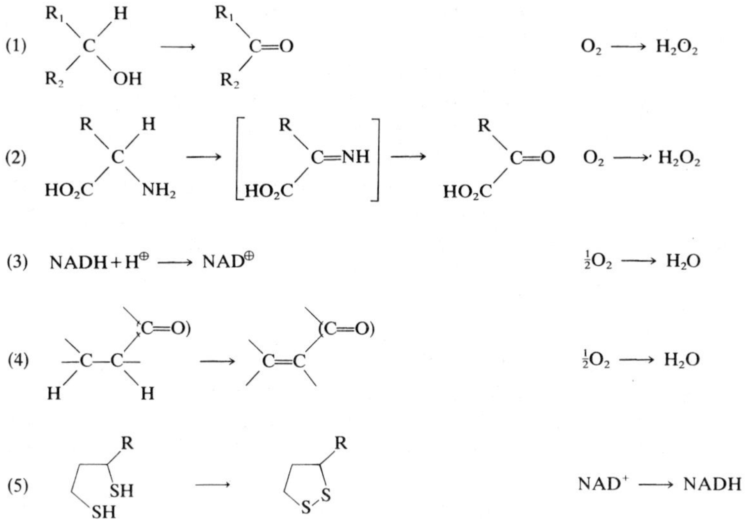

SCHEME 6.14

oxygen to give hydrogen peroxide, whereas the reoxidation takes place indirectly through the medium of an electron transport system in the case of reactions (3) and (4). In the last example NAD^+ acts as acceptor of hydrogen and the cycle as a whole shows how FAD mediates in the reoxidation of dihydrolipoic acid at the expense of NAD^+ (cf. Scheme 5.15 in the last chapter). One striking feature of these cycles is the ability of the dihydroflavin to transfer hydrogen to molecular oxygen, an ability not shared with the nicotinamide coenzymes. In reacting with oxygen in this way the flavins perform a vital service as will be explained later.

Mechanism of action

In embarking on a survey of the mechanism of action of the flavin coenzymes we encounter once again an unsolved problem that is currently the subject of very active research. This aspect of flavin biochemistry is bedevilled by the same combination of circumstances which complicate the issue in the case of the nicotinamides: a diverse range of reactions, matched by a welter of mechanistic theories but with, so far, few hard experimental facts to provide a firm basis for discussion. Many different reactions are under active investigation at the present time but in this account we shall again concentrate on just one, the oxidation of an alcohol to a carbonyl derivative, reaction (1) in Scheme 6.14, and it has been selected for no better reason than the desire to have a direct comparison between the subject matter of this section and that of the earlier section dealing with the mechanism of action of the nicotinamide coenzymes.

The reaction is shown in more detail in Scheme 6.15. Two different hydrogens are transferred from the substrate, one from carbon and the other from oxygen, but in this case the destination of each hydrogen in the coenzyme cannot be determined by isotopic labelling experiments, because in the dihydroflavin both hydrogens are susceptible to exchange with the medium. Therefore, the direction of attack specified in the following mechanistic schemes represents a purely arbitrary choice and in each case there is an equally plausible alternative involving initial attack at the second site of hydrogen addition. From the electronic point of view, the reaction mechanisms can be classified on the same basis as that adopted in the section on the nicotinamides, that is, according to the type of cleavage which takes place in the C-H bond of the substrate. In principle this could lead to transfer of a hydride, a hydrogen atom, a proton, or as a final possibility the cleavage might be part of a pericyclic process. This time three possible mechanisms are given to show how this key step might take place. The first two show transfer of a hydride (Scheme 6.16) or a hydrogen atom (Scheme 6.17). They are directly comparable to the equivalent mechanisms advanced in the case of the nicotinamides and therefore will not be discussed in detail. In the third mechanism (Scheme 6.18) the substrate combines with the flavin residue in a standard nucleophilic addition and the oxidation takes place in the second step by means of a fragmentation. In this mechanism, first proposed by Hamilton, all the hydrogens are transferred as *protons*. From what has been said already, it will be apparent that the true mechanism is not known, and all we can do is briefly examine the available evidence to see how far it can be accommodated within these schemes.

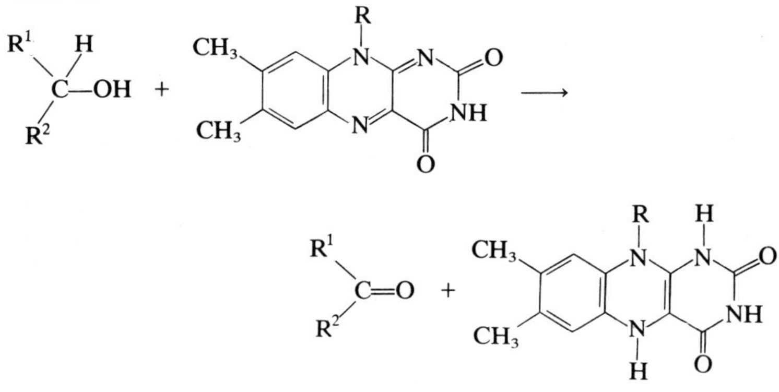

SCHEME 6.15

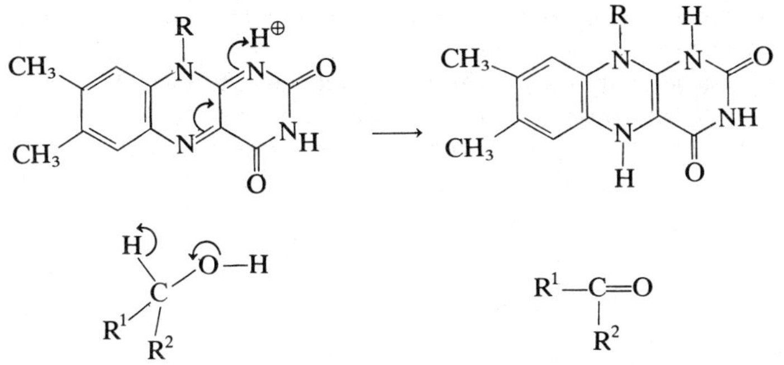

SCHEME 6.16

Simple model flavins readily undergo a redox change, analogous to that of the coenzyme, with a variety of reagents, and there is unequivocal proof that, under certain conditions, these reactions involve the formation of a radical intermediate, probably a semiquinone radical of the type shown in Scheme 6.17. The intermediate can be detected by characteristic changes in the light absorption spectrum and it shows the expected signal in the e.s.r. spectrum. Similar characteristic changes in the visible spectrum have been observed for certain enzymic reactions but puzzlingly they are not always accompanied by the signal in the e.s.r. spectrum. In order to accommodate these conflicting results it has been

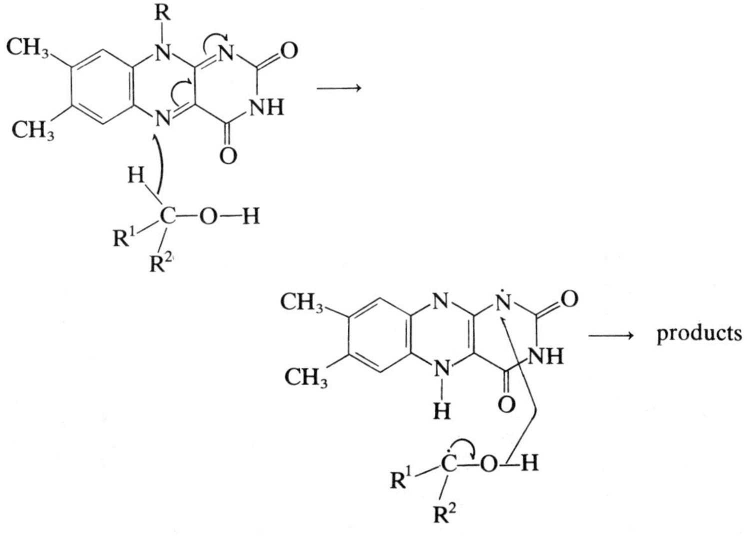

SCHEME 6.17

suggested that a semiquinone radical is indeed formed, but that it may be prevented from giving an e.s.r. signal by interaction with a neighbouring thiol residue on the enzyme. Thus the situation is fluid and it is probable that flavin coenzymes may react by either a free radical mechanism or a two-electron mechanism depending on the particular enzyme and substrate.

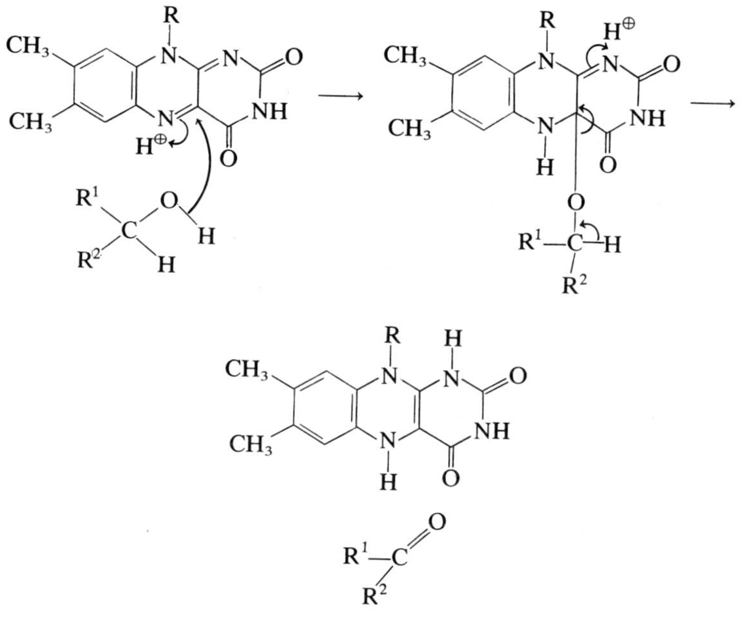

SCHEME 6.18

The nicotinamides and flavins: a comparison of metabolic role

It is interesting to compare the function of the two classes of coenzyme which mediate in hydrogen transfer in the light of what is known about their mechanism of action, because the nicotinamides and the flavins are employed in significantly different roles. We have already seen how the nicotinamides function in effect as vehicles of hydrogen transport, carrying hydrogen from those reactions in which a substrate is oxidized to others in which a substrate is reduced. In this way each nicotinamide coenzyme provides a medium for exchange of hydrogen which is accessible to a vast range of enzymes and metabolites, and the arrangement results in a simpler and more economical mode of operation. Thus each metabolite only requires one enzyme to draw hydrogen from the pool, or to donate hydrogen to it as the case may be, and in principle a particular reaction may take place at the expense of the oxidation or reduction of any one of a whole range of metabolites. Obviously the alternative mode of operation, direct transfer of hydrogen from metabolite to metabolite, would require a vastly greater number of enzymes to achieve the same flexibility of operation.

The flavins, on the other hand, operate in a much more restricted way: a typical flavoprotein will accept hydrogen from a specific metabolite and will then be oxidized by a specific oxidant, so that, although the hydrogen transfer takes place via the flavin, it is the equivalent of a direct transfer of hydrogen from one substrate to another in its mode of operation. On this basis it might be supposed that the organization of metabolism could be streamlined by replacing the existing enzymes based on the flavin system by equivalent enzymes based on the nicotinamides. However, this supposition fails to take into account the special character of the reaction cycles in which the flavoproteins mediate as agents of hydrogen transfer. Almost always the reoxidation step is carried out either directly or indirectly by molecular oxygen. This special ability of the flavin to undergo redox reactions with molecular oxygen (and also with metal ions as we shall see later) allows them to fill a vital role.

Thus molecular oxygen is normally the ultimate source of oxidizing power available to those cells which derive their energy from the oxidative degradation of organic materials. However, the direct reaction of oxygen with a typical organic metabolite is exceptionally difficult to achieve in the medium of a living cell, even though there will usually be a very favourable free-energy change associated with the desired reaction. This barrier to direct reaction may be unfortunate in one sense but it is providential in another, for without it living systems as we know them would be liable to spontaneous combustion in the earth's atmosphere, and life as we know it would not be possible.

The reason for this kinetic barrier to reaction lies in the structure of the oxygen molecule. Molecular oxygen exists as a triplet (i.e. the diradical form $\cdot O\!-\!O\cdot$), and therefore readily takes part in reactions which involve the movement of unpaired electrons (typically radical reactions or redox reactions with metal ions), but not in reactions which would involve movement of paired electrons. On the other hand, a typical organic compound exists in the singlet state (all electrons paired), and is therefore prone to react by a mechanism in which the electrons remain paired. It does not react readily by a one-electron mechanism, unless there is a special structural feature in the molecule which can stabilize a radical intermediate.

The cell commonly employs a flavoprotein as intermediary to overcome this barrier to direct reaction between oxygen and an organic substrate. We have already seen that the flavin nucleus has the potential to undergo redox reactions by either a one-electron mechanism or by a mechanism in which all the electrons remain paired. Presumably the flavin can abstract hydrogen from the organic substrate by a paired electron mechanism (as in Scheme 6.16 or 6.17), and can then switch to a radical mechanism in the reaction with molecular oxygen (see Scheme 6.19). In contrast the nicotinamide system does not show this capacity to react by a radical mechanism in enzymic reactions or equivalent model reactions.

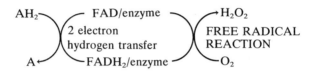

SCHEME 6.19

This flexibility of mechanism is probably exploited throughout the range of flavin-mediated hydrogen transfers. For example, in the reoxidation of dihydrolipoic acid, reaction (5) in Scheme 6.14, NAD^+ rather than molecular oxygen acts as reoxidant, and therefore this step probably does not involve a radical mechanism. However, the first step of the process is also atypical in that hydrogen is abstracted from sulphur rather than carbon and there is evidence that it may go by a radical mechanism. So again, the flavin probably undergoes a switch of mechanism between one redox reaction and the other.

The great importance of this flexibility of reaction of the flavin nucleus is reflected in the evolution of a large number of highly specialized flavoproteins. For example, in some flavoproteins (called metalloflavoproteins) the flavin residue appears to act in cooperation with an enzyme-bound metal ion. The metal possibly assists in the overall redox reaction by accepting electrons from the reduced flavin and then passing them on to the acceptor. Such redox reactions with metals are commonly one-electron transfers (e.g. $Fe^{III} \rightarrow Fe^{II}$) and in them we see yet another way in which the flexible reactivity of the flavin nucleus can be exploited.

Finally, it should be mentioned that flavoproteins are employed to bring about transformations quite different from the straightforward hydrogen transfers discussed so far. An example is given in Scheme 6.20 where an organic substrate is hydroxylated by what amounts to the insertion of an oxygen atom derived from molecular oxygen into a C–H bond. The second atom of the oxygen molecule is reduced to water by

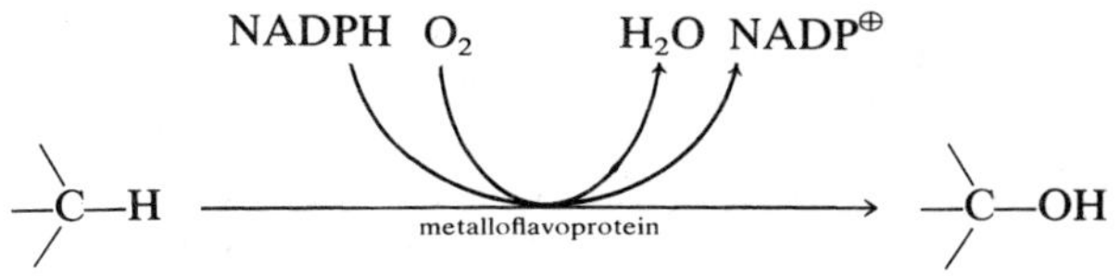

NADPH O$_2$ H$_2$O NADP$^{\oplus}$

$$-\overset{|}{\underset{|}{C}}-H \xrightarrow[\text{metalloflavoprotein}]{} -\overset{|}{\underset{|}{C}}-OH$$

SCHEME 6.20

means of hydrogen derived from NADPH. This remarkable reaction hinges on the metalloflavoprotein component. It is without parallel in standard organic chemical practice although some of the catalytic oxygenation reactions employed in the petrochemical industry may well be related in mechanism. The process has been the subject of both speculation and investigation but it is beyond the scope of this book to delve any deeper into the topic.

To summarize, it can be stated that, despite much research, the mechanism of action of both the nicotinamide and flavin coenzymes is still completely open, and this area of investigation represents one of the major challenges waiting for the chemist who is interested in investigating the mechanism of biological reactions.

7. The electron transport system

HAVING digressed from the theme of bioenergetics in the last chapter, we now return to it with a detailed consideration of the mechanics of the electron transport system. In the introductory survey of metabolism in Chapter 1 it was explained that this system operates in effect as an accessory to a number of catabolic pathways, and it makes its contribution by carrying out two separate, though closely interdependent, functions. Firstly, it provides the means of oxidation at the appropriate steps of the various pathways, either directly by reaction with the metabolite as in the conversion of succinic acid to fumaric acid, or indirectly by recycling NADH to NAD$^+$. Secondly, it brings about the regeneration of ATP from its hydrolysis products, by harnessing the energy released in the various processes of oxidation. It was in recognition of this latter role, oxidative phosphorylation, that the electron transport system was dubbed the power station of the cell, and in examining the mechanics of the process we reach the climax of our survey of bioenergetics.

At the outset, it must be admitted that the mode of operation of the system as a whole is still shrouded in mystery. The problem is under very active investigation on many fronts and all we can do in this brief treatment is to summarize the present state of knowledge and to consider the merits of some current theories on the mechanism of action. As we shall see, some aspects of the problem are still totally baffling, while others appear to be tantalizingly close to solution.

The organization of the electron transport system

The system is of breathtaking complexity in both the chemical and the biological sense, and it is desirable to begin with a brief outline of its cell biology so that the chemical aspects, to be discussed later, will be seen in a more meaningful perspective. The active components of the system are not free to diffuse throughout the interior of the cell but are located in a special compartment. In bacterial cells this structure is located on the wall of the cell, whereas in the cells of other organisms such as mammals it takes the form of a specially adapted sub-cellular particle (or granule) called the mitochondrion, and a given cell may contain several hundreds of these minute bodies. In the interests of brevity, we will only survey the properties of mitochondrial electron transport systems and will not take into account the important differences shown by the bacterial system. The mitochondrion is a sausage-shaped body, enclosed by a lipid membrane (i.e. a membrane based on long-chain aliphatic hydrocarbons). The interior is sub-divided by further lipid membranes to which most of the active components of the electron transport system appear to be attached. The components appear to be grouped in carefully ordered repeating units in which each component has a defined orientation with respect to its neighbours. Thus the interior of the mitochondrion is cut off from the general medium of the cell and it provides what is in effect a carefully regulated reaction vessel for the operation of the electron transport system (and other processes).

Intact mitochondria can be separated from the assorted contents of the cell after rupture of the cell-wall (typically of liver cells). When isolated under carefully controlled conditions the mitochondria are viable, and, given a supply of the necessary materials (including NADH, oxygen, ADP, and inorganic phosphate), they will readily carry out the normal processes of the electron transport system.

The next stage of the investigation is to disrupt the mitochondrion itself under more vigourous conditions, so that the individual active components are detached from the membrane, with the aim of isolating them for individual study in solution. Unfortunately, this operation usually requires relatively drastic physical or chemical methods of disruption with the consequent risk of damage to the delicate components under study. A second difficulty arises from the fact that even if a particular component survives isolation without suffering significant structural damage, it may exhibit properties in aqueous solution that differ markedly from those it possesses in the specialized, probably hydrophobic, environment of the mitochondrial membrane where it normally operates. Thirdly, there is evidence that the normal functioning of the electron transport system depends critically on the spatial arrangement of the individual components, and, inevitably, this vital orientation of one component with respect to another will be lost after the components have been removed from the membrane. Finally, there is a strong possibility that the membrane itself may play an active part in the overall process. In the face of all these difficulties it is not surprising that the working of the electron transport system still defies solution and the considerable progress that has been achieved so far represents a remarkable triumph of experimental skill.

It is convenient to divide the treatment of the electron transport system into two separate sections, the first dealing with the chemistry of the redox reactions and the second with the phenomenon of oxidative phosphorylation. This line of attack will be adopted in the following account.

The redox reactions

The role of the respiratory chain

Some typical oxidations brought about by the mitochondrion with the assistance of the electron transport system are shown in Scheme 7.1. The first two take place in the electron transport system itself and they will be considered in detail in this account. The third shows the dehydrogenation of a fatty acid derivative which is one of the steps of fatty acid catabolism. This process involves the electron transport system in a less direct way and so it will not be considered in detail until Chapter 10.

(1) $NADH \longrightarrow NAD^+$

(2)

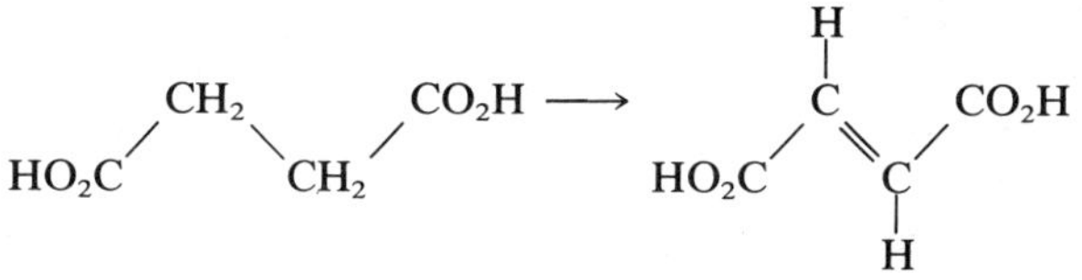

(3)

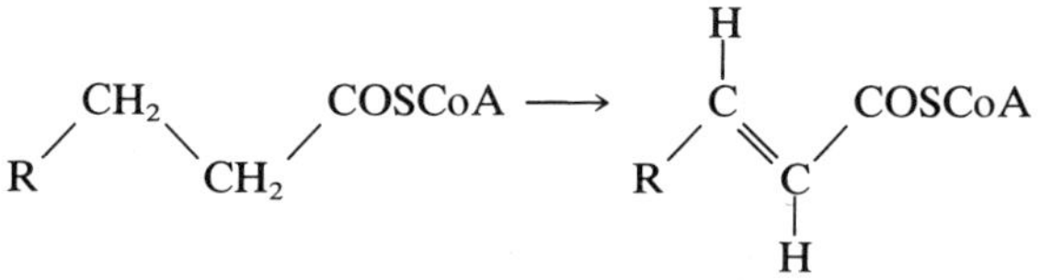

SCHEME 7.1. Oxidations in the mitochondria.

Although the overall process corresponds in each case to the dehydrogenation of an organic molecule at the expense of molecular oxygen, it is clear that direct reaction between the substrate and oxygen is not involved. Instead a chain of redox reactions intervenes, in which one component reduces the next, until, at the end of the chain, oxygen is reduced to water. The phenomenon is usually referred to as electron transport and the general pattern of operation for a chain involving components A, B, C, etc. is shown in Scheme 7.2. Each component cycles between the oxidized (ox) and reduced (red) forms and in the context of the electron transport system the device as a whole is usually referred to as the respiratory chain. In the investigation of the electron transport system much effort has been devoted to the isolation of these components and those that have been characterized to date are discussed in turn below.

The components of the respiratory chain

Flavoproteins. Several different flavoprotein components have been isolated from mitochondria and it is probable that they play a part in the

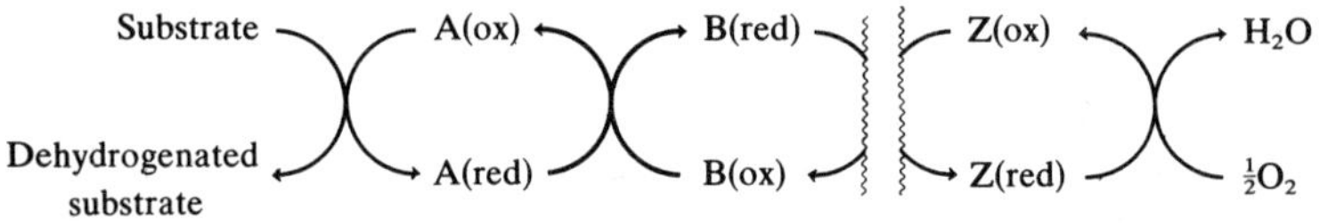

SCHEME 7.2

process of electron transport by cycling between the fully oxidized and fully reduced (dihydro) forms. As we shall see later, a flavoprotein probably serves as the first component of the chain and a separate flavoprotein is required for each of the different organic substrates.

Ubiquinones. These comprize a family of compounds which have the general structure [55], in which a quinonoid ring is attached to a long isoprenoid side-chain. It is thought that the operative part of the molecule is the quinone ring which can take part in the chain of redox reactions by cycling between the quinone and the corresponding dihydro compound (ubiquinol), [56]. Ubiquinones can be extracted from intact mitochondria simply by washing them with organic solvents. Such deficient mitochondria show a reduction in their ability to carry out their characteristic oxidative reactions but the normal level of activity can be restored simply by returning an adequate supply of ubiquinone to the system. On this basis it is assumed that unlike the other components the ubiquinones are not structurally bound to the lipid membrane but are effectively dissolved in it. No doubt the long hydrocarbon side-chain plays its part by endowing the molecules with the necessary solubility characteristics to ensure that they remain associated with the hydrophobic environment of membrane. The ubiquinones are clearly free to diffuse through the membrane and it is possible that this mobility is exploited in some way in the operation of the electron transport system.

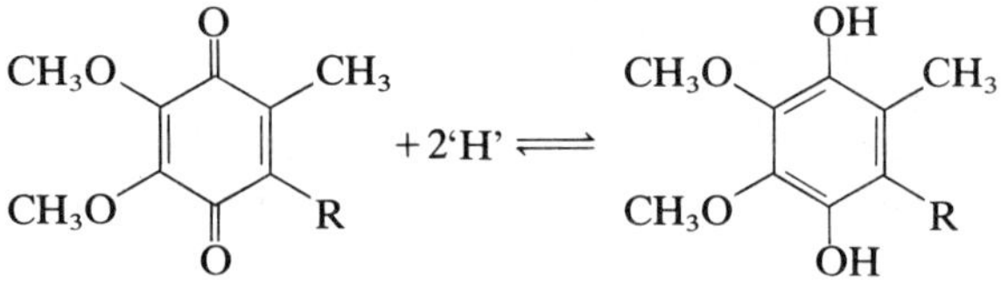

Ubiquinone   Ubiquinol
[55]   [56]

$$R = -(CH_2CH=\overset{\overset{\displaystyle CH_3}{|}}{C}-CH_2)_n H; \quad n \leqslant 10$$

Cytochromes. These comprise a second family of structurally related components and the individual members of the series are designated on a trivial basis (from the standpoint of the electron transport system) by subscripts such as a, a_1 or b. They are bonded to the membrane and disruptive methods are required for their isolation.

Each cytochrome has at its core an iron atom bound in a porphyrin ring, as in [57]. The iron is hexacoordinate, the fifth and sixth ligands being provided by the protein matrix in which the porphyrin ring is embedded. The metal atom acts as a redox agent by cycling between the Fe^{III} and Fe^{II} states. In each cytochrome the iron has a characteristic redox potential, E_0', which changes markedly through the series from 0·075 V in cytochrome b to 0·29 V in cytochrome a. (The redox potential, E_0', is measured under standardized conditions at pH 7.) Presumably this variation results from the change in the environment of the metal in the different compounds.

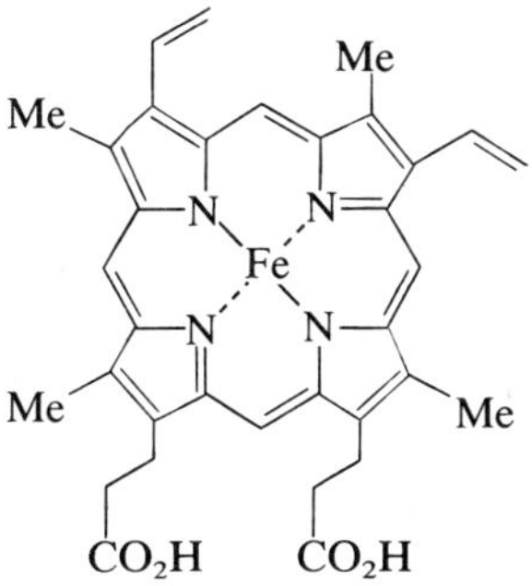

[57]

This completes the list of components which have been reliably characterized but it must be borne in mind that there may be other active components too unstable to survive the rigours of the currently available methods of isolation.

Order of components in the chain

It is assumed that these components cooperate in the redox transfers by forming a respiratory chain following the pattern shown in Scheme 7.2. It is generally supposed that the components will come into play in the order of increasing value of E_0', and the currently favoured sequence of operation in the case of NADH oxidation is shown in Scheme 7.3; the value of E_0' corresponding to each component is listed alongside. However it must be borne in mind that the redox potentials/shown in the list are those measured for the isolated components, and so, for the reasons mentioned earlier, the sequence must be regarded as no more than a tentative proposal. (Note that cytochrome b is out or order. Its position in the chain is an open question.)

Scheme 7.4 shows the corresponding sequence proposed for the oxidation of succinic acid. With the exception of the first stage, which takes place on a different flavoprotein, the chain is identical with that proposed for NADH. Thus, in the overall plan it is envisaged that each substrate would be dehydrogenated on its corresponding flavoprotein, with ubiquinone acting as acceptor; the resulting ubiquinol would then diffuse via the membrane to a neighbouring chain of cytochromes where it would be reoxidized at the expense of molecular oxygen.

This working hypothesis has received support from recent experiments in which mitochondria were disrupted under conditions carefully controlled so as to be sufficiently vigorous to produce partial cleavage of the membrane, but avoiding complete disruption of the respiratory chains. The resulting mixture of fragments can be fractionated according to the nature of the active components, and so far four active fractions, designated complexes I, II, III, and IV, have been separated. Their constitution is indicated in Scheme 7.4 and the corresponding sites of cleavage are marked by dotted lines. Taken together, the four complexes contain all the known components of the respiratory chains involved in the oxidation of NADH and succinic acid, apart from cytochrome c and ubiquinone (which is mobile in any case). It is reassuring to note that the

	E_0' (V)
NADH	-0.32
$\downarrow$	
Flavoprotein	$0 \leqslant -0.18$ (value uncertain)
$\downarrow$	
Ubiquinone	$+0.098$
$\downarrow$	
Cytochrome b (Cyt b)	$+0.075$
$\downarrow$	
Cytochrome c_1	$+0.22$
$\downarrow$	
Cytochrome c	$+0.25$
$\downarrow$	
Cytochrome $(a + a_3)$	$+0.29$
$\downarrow$	
O_2/H_2O	$+0.82$

SCHEME 7.3. Order of components in the respiratory chain.

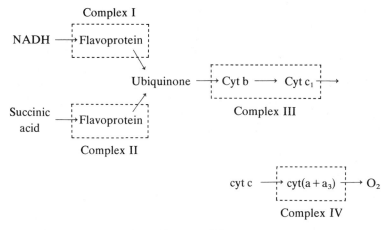

SCHEME 7.4

composition and behaviour of the individual complexes is in accord with the proposed sequence shown in Scheme 7.3. Thus complex I will affect the oxidation of NADH to NAD^+ using a compound of the ubiquinone class as hydrogen acceptor; complex II will dehydrogenate succinic acid under similar conditions; ubiquinol will reduce cytochrome c ($Fe^{III} \rightarrow Fe^{II}$) in the presence of complex III; finally, in the presence of complex IV, the reduced form of cytochrome c will bring about the reduction of oxygen to water. Moreover, by combining the appropriate complexes with a supply of cytochrome c and a suitable ubiquinone, it is possible to produce mixtures that have the ability to carry out the dehydrogenation of NADH or succinic acid, the final step in each case being the reduction of oxygen to water.

Mechanism of the redox reactions

The isolation of these complexes represents an exciting breakthrough for it is now possible to study the mechanism of the redox reactions that take place in the different sections of the redox chain, in isolation from the whole. This is a very rapidly developing area of research and as yet no clear picture has emerged. Therefore in this account we will do no more than survey some of the major questions which are under active investigation.

Obviously there is the problem of electronic mechanism for each of the redox reactions taking place in the respiratory chain. Presumably the reactions in the cytochrome section of the chain will take place by a mechanism involving transfer of one electron, for in each case the metal ion cycles between the Fe^{III} and Fe^{II} states. On the other hand, the first step in which NADH or succinic acid transfers hydrogen to a flavin, will probably take place by a mechanism in which the electrons remain paired (e.g. transfer of a hydride ion followed by a proton), for reasons explained in the last chapter. That being so, there would need to be, at some stage, a component which effects the switch from one type of mechanism to the other. Possible candidates for this key role are the flavoprotein or the ubiquinone for both have the potential to undergo a redox reaction by either class of mechanism. This switch of mechanism may be of more than academic interest because it is possibly bound up with the process of oxidative phosphorylation as we shall see later.

Assuming that it can be shown that the redox reactions taking place in the cytochrome section of the chain involve the transfer of electrons one at a time, there is still the puzzling problem of how the electron can be transferred from one metal ion to the next. In each cytochrome the metal is buried inside a protein sheath and therefore it is difficult to conceive how electron transfer can take place by direct contact of the Fe^{III} ion of one cytochrome with the Fe^{II} ion of the next. To overcome this difficulty it has been proposed that one or more groups on the protein itself might be actively involved in transporting the electron from the outside of the protein sheath to the metal ion on the inside. One possible candidate for this role would be a thiol group which could ferry electrons by cycling between a thiol and a sulphur radical. Presumably the group would be able to move from the surface of the cytochrome structure to a position adjacent to the metal ion on the inside, possibly as the consequence of a conformational change in the protein sheath. An alternative proposal envisages the electron being conducted via the π-bonds of one or more suitably aligned aryl rings. The aromatic systems of the normal amino acids tyrosine, phenylalanine, or tryptophan could serve in this way, as could the π-system of the porphyrin ring itself.

Finally, at the end of the respiratory chain, the reduction of oxygen to water poses an intriguing mechanistic problem. Overall the molecule of oxygen combines with four electrons and four protons to generate two molecules of water. The electrons are delivered via the cytochrome chain and therefore they may be presumed to be transfered to the oxygen molecule one at a time. However, no intermediates corresponding to partial reduction of oxygen (such as H_2O_2) have been detected as yet, and so it is not clear how the reduction of oxygen takes place. In this connection it is interesting that the complex which carries out the transformation contains copper as well as iron, and it would not be surprising if copper turns out to be the active agent that reduces oxygen in this key step.

Thus the mechanistic problems posed by the redox reactions of the respiratory chain are both varied and extraordinarily complex. Nevertheless, steady progress is being made on several fronts and hopefully we will not have to wait long for the answers to some of these questions.

Oxidative phosphorylation

The coupling of oxidation to phosphorylation

Having covered the chemistry of the redox reactions we are now in a position to consider the equally fascinating problem posed by the process of oxidative phosphorylation. At the outset it must be admitted that we can hardly begin to explain the phenomenon in terms of a chemical mechanism. In this account we shall survey what little information has been obtained from experiments on both the biological system and model compounds. We shall also assess the merits of various theories that have been advanced but as we shall see, this vital aspect of metabolism is still a complete mystery.

As mentioned earlier, oxidative phosphorylation takes place efficiently in intact isolated mitochondria: that is, when they are provided with a supply of NAD (or other suitable substrate), molecular oxygen, ADP and inorganic phosphate, mitochondria can oxidize the substrate and at the same time generate ATP. By measuring the rate of turnover for the two reactions it is possible to show that approximately three moles of ATP are generated for each mole of NADH consumed. This relationship is a key one and it is commonly designated the P/O ratio, that is, the ratio of phosphate conversion to oxygen consumption. The P/O ratio for the oxidation of succinic acid is only 2, as opposed to the value of 3 for NADH, and in this connection it is interesting that, with oxygen as terminal acceptor, considerably more free energy is available from the oxidation of NADH to NAD^+ (220 kJ mol^{-1}) than is liberated in the dehydrogenation of succinic acid to fumaric acid (160 kJ mol^{-1}).

Under normal conditions in freshly isolated mitochondria, the two processes of oxidation and phosphorylation appear to be tightly coupled. For example, it is possible to reduce the rate of the oxidation process by limiting the supply of ADP or inorganic phosphate, even when NADH and oxygen are in abundant supply. However, this tight coupling only holds in freshly isolated mitochondria. After isolation a steady deterioration takes place accompanied by swelling of the structure and a steady fall in the observed P/O ratio. More strikingly still, the coupling of the two reactions can be suspended completely by adding a variety of simple compounds to the medium. For example, in the presence of 2,4-dinitrophenol, mitochondria will rapidly oxidize NADH without giving rise to any apparent net synthesis of ATP. The coupling of the two reactions can be restored, however, simply by removing the phenol, so the electron transport system does not suffer irreversible damage as a consequence of the uncoupling process. It is not clear how the 2,4-dinitrophenol achieves its effect. Thus, although it may truly uncouple the two reactions in the sense that the oxidation of NADH proceeds without ATP being formed, it is equally possible that it could produce the observed effect merely by bringing about the immediate hydrolysis of any ATP synthesized in the normal way.

Mechanism of the coupling

From these results it would appear that the two processes of oxidation and phosphorylation are closely linked, at least under normal conditions of operation. Many ingenious theories have been advanced to account for this phenomenon. Although they vary widely in detail they can be grouped according to their principle of operation into the three categories discussed in turn below.

Chemical coupling. The proposals which come under this heading have as their common characteristic the two processes chemically linked by means of a common intermediate. In general it is envisaged that a phosphoryl residue might be combined chemically with one of the components of the respiratory chain. This (low-energy) phosphate derivative would then be converted by oxidation to one of high energy which would in turn drive the formation of ATP by transfer of a phosphoryl group to ADP in the usual way.

We have already met in Chapter 3 an example of ATP formation outside the electron transport system which relies for its effect on this strategy. The sequence of reactions is shown in Scheme 7.5 and it forms part of the pathway of glucose catabolism. Its mechanism is relevant to the present discussion because it achieves its effect by chemically coupling an oxidative reaction to a phosphorylation, so that the energy released in the former transformation is harnessed to drive the latter.

In the first step the level of oxidation at C-2 is raised from that of an alcohol to the equivalent of a ketone and as a consequence the low-energy phosphate derative [58] is converted to the key high-energy phosphate, phosphoenol pyruvate [59]. Note that the redox reaction takes place internally so that the oxidation at C-2 takes place at

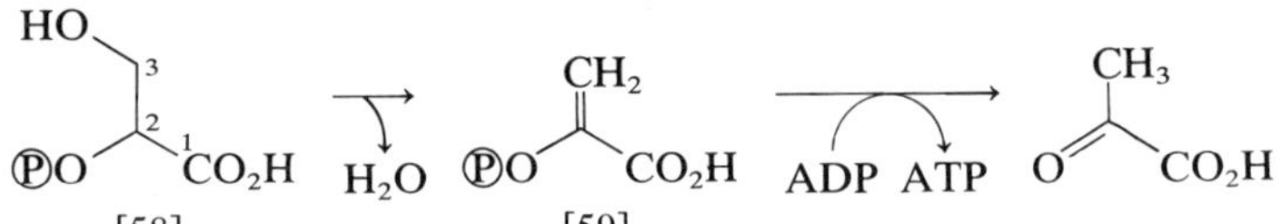

SCHEME 7.5

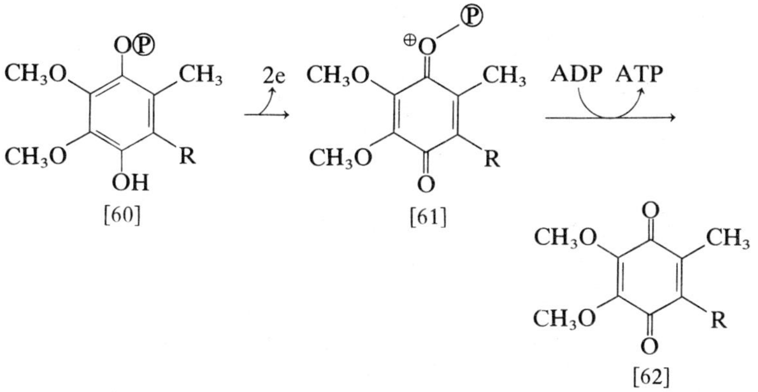

Scheme 7.6

the expense of a reduction at C-1. However, even though the molecule as a whole is not oxidized the essential point remains: a phosphate derivative with a low potential for phosphoryl group transfer is converted to one of high potential simply by raising the oxidation level at the carbon to which the phosphate group is attached.

A number of schemes have been advanced to show how the redox reactions of the respiratory chain might be coupled in an equivalent way to the regeneration of ATP. Only one will be considered here, and in it a ubiquinone serves as the common agent of electron transfer and oxidative phosphorylation. The key steps of the proposal are shown in Scheme 7.6 in which we see the quinol phosphate, [60] being oxidized by one of the components of the respiratory chain to an unstable quinoid intermediate [61]. The phosphate group in [61] would be expected to be extremely susceptible to nucleophilic attack, and, in the electron transport system, the formation of ATP would be brought about by attack of the terminal phosphate residue of ADP. No direct evidence in support of the proposed scheme has come from investigations of the electron transport system itself, but the chemical feasibility of the process has been established by means of the simple model reaction shown in Scheme 7.7. The formation of pyrophosphate in this model reaction provides a particularly persuasive analogy for ATP formation in the mitochondrion.

In the biological process the quinone, [62] would have to be recycled to the quinol phosphate [60]. Apart from the formation of the phosphate link, this reaction sequence would have to include a reduction step and this would be effected by the preceding member of the respiratory chain.

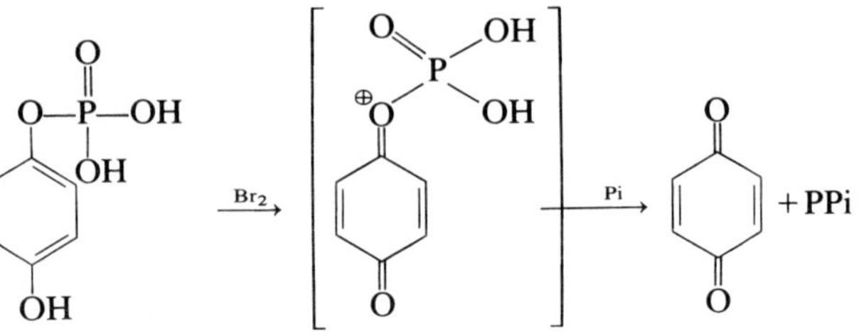

SCHEME 7.7

Equivalent cycles have been proposed in which other components act as the agent of oxidative phosphorylation but since there is no experimental evidence to support any of them, they will not be discussed in detail.

Apart from achieving the phosphorylation of ADP, the cycle, whatever its nature, would provide a vehicle for the indirect transfer of two electrons (or two hydrogens depending on the mechanism) between successive components of the respiratory chain, and the free energy to drive the cycle would be derived from the overall redox reaction between these two components. Therefore, in order to achieve a useful net synthesis of ATP, the redox process would have to provide a minimum of, say, 35 kJ mol^{-1}. This free-energy change corresponds to a difference in redox potential of about 0·18 V for a reaction which takes place by the transfer of two electrons or their equivalent, or 0·09 V for one which involves the transfer of one electron. Naturally, in the latter case the redox reaction would need to operate twice for each turn of the phosphorylation cycle.

On this basis only three steps of the respiratory chain leading from NADH to oxygen would qualify for consideration (see Scheme 7.3); firstly, the transfer of two hydrogens from NADH to the corresponding flavoprotein (estimated to yield between 30 and 60 kJ mol^{-1}); secondly, the transfer of electrons from cytochrome b to cytochrome c (equivalent to a two-electron transfer yielding 35 kJ mol^{-1}); and thirdly, the reduction of oxygen by the final cytochrome (on the same basis equivalent to a yield of 100 kJ mol^{-1}). We have already seen that three units of ATP are generated for each mole of NADH converted to NAD$^+$, so on the basis of chemical coupling it is reasonable to expect that there should be three separate sites of ATP formation. Indeed it is often pointed out that such an arrangement would provide a rationale for the complex character of the respiratory chain: thus a multi-stage sequence of transfer would ensure that the energy is released in discrete packets instead of all at once and in this way it would facilitate the generation of more than one unit of ATP for each molecule of substrate undergoing oxidation.

Further circumstantial evidence that oxidative phosphorylation is chemically coupled to specific steps of the respiratory chain comes from the observation that only two molecules of ATP are generated as a consequence of succinic acid oxidation. In this connection it is significant that the transfer of hydrogen from succinic acid to its corresponding flavoprotein releases very little energy and therefore this step, unlike the corresponding step in the chain leading from NADH, would not have the potential to drive ATP formation. However it must be emphasized once again that there is no direct evidence in favour of chemical coupling from studies on the electron transport system itself: no unusual phosphory-lated intermediates have been detected, and although isolated fragments of the respiratory chain will carry out the appropriate redox reactions, there is no evidence that ATP is generated as a consequence.

Chemiosmotic coupling. A particularly striking feature of the mitochondrion is its carefully ordered structure in which the interior is closely sub-divided into separate compartments by lipid membranes. It is already clear that these membranes make an important contribution to the working of the electron transport system, by providing the framework on which the components can be organized into coherent chains. However, the membrane may not be confined to this passive role and, in view of the total lack of support for a chemical mechanism of coupling, it becomes increasingly likely that the membrane may play an active part in bringing about the coupling of ATP formation to the redox reactions.

Two schemes based on this possibility will be considered. The first will be discussed in this section, and it rests on the supposition that the protons and hydroxide ions generated as by-products of the redox reactions may hold the key to oxidative phosphorylation. The hydroxide ions are formed at the end of the respiratory chain when oxygen is reduced as in Scheme 7.8. These are balanced by the release of four protons at an earlier stage. The precise timing of proton release is not known but presumbaly it would take place at the stage where the mechanism of the redox reactions switches from transfer of hydrogen to transfer of electrons. This point is illustrated for the reoxidation of a quinol by transfer of electrons in Scheme 7.9.

Since two such events would take place for each molecule of oxygen undergoing reduction, the system as a whole remains in balance and in principle the protons can combine with the hydroxide ions to form water.

$$2H_2O + O_2 \xrightarrow{\;4e\;} 4OH^{\ominus}$$

SCHEME 7.8

However, in the fully operational electron transport system the redox reactions take place under tightly controlled conditions in the environment of the mitochondrion, and it is conceivable that the protons may be liberated in one compartment and the hydroxide ions in another. Furthermore, if the two sets of ions are prevented from migrating freely between the two compartments by the membrane which separates them (a reasonable property to expect of a membrane), then a potential energy gradient will be set up across the membrane as a consequence of the redox reactions. According to the chemiosmotic theory, this would provide the driving force for ATP formation in the mitochondrion. It is envisaged that a special device would allow the assisted passage of the trapped protons across the membrane and this controlled migration would be coupled to ATP formation. It is beyond the scope of this book to discuss how this might be achieved in practice but there are reasonably close precedents for the proposed behaviour among the known properties of biological membranes.

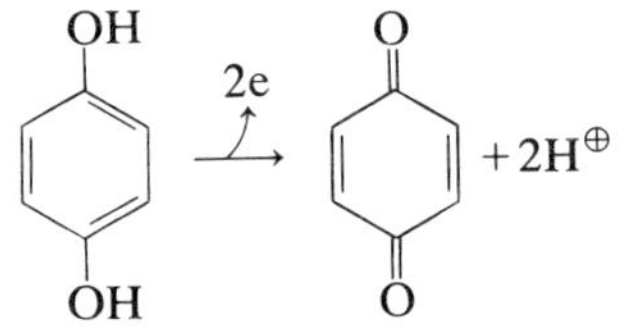

$$\underset{\text{OH}}{\overset{\text{OH}}{\bigodot}} \xrightarrow{2e} \underset{\text{O}}{\overset{\text{O}}{\bigodot}} + 2\text{H}^{\oplus}$$

SCHEME 7.9

Mechanical Coupling. This scheme also invokes a specialized role for the mitochondrial membrane in the transfer of the free energy from the redox reactions to the process by which ATP is generated. No detailed scheme has been formulated but, in general terms, it is envisaged that the energy would be transmitted mechanically from one reaction site to the other by a conformational change in the membrane structure.

Unfortunately there is no direct evidence to show that the mitochondrial membrane possesses the special properties required for either chemiosmotic coupling or mechanical coupling and therefore the mechanism of oxidative phosphorylation remains a total mystery. However, given the enormous interest in the problem, and the considerable effort being devoted to its solution, it seems reasonable to hope for a decisive breakthrough in the not too distant future.

8. The pathway of glucose catabolism

THE POLICY followed so far in this book has been to study different types of reaction one by one in separate chapters. This approach has the advantage that it is possible to present a coherent treatment of the chemistry and biochemistry of the selected reactions. Unfortunately, however, an important perspective is lacking in this approach and on its own it cannot lead to a full understanding of the chemical basis of metabolism.

This missing perspective relates to the detailed organization of the metabolic pathways (all we have seen so far is outline schemes showing general strategy). In order to make good the deficiency the next three chapters will be devoted to a step by step analysis of a selection of metabolic pathways. In each case the analysis will have three facets: firstly, the energetics of the pathway; secondly, its preparative strategy; and thirdly, the mechanisms of the reactions involved (where they have not been covered already).

After a brief introduction each pathway will be presented in a standard schematic form in which the reactions will run down the left side of the page with a commentary running in parallel on the right. This commentary is intended to draw attention to any point of interest concerning the mechanism or energetics of the individual steps, but in order to keep the schemes compact and easy to follow, the comments will be kept as brief as possible; where necessary they will be amplified in the subsequent discussion.

The pathway of glucose catabolism is the obvious place to begin. Its general importance throughout the biosphere has been amply stressed in earlier chapters and the total annual turnover of the reactions concerned must reach staggering proportions.

In Chapter 1 it was explained that the pathway is divided into two stages as indicated in Scheme 8.1 and it is appropriate to start by elaborating on the reasons for this division. First, both pyruvic acid and acetyl CoA represent branch points at which other pathways feed material into the pathway under consideration (or siphon material off as the case may be). Consequently, although the steps of glycolysis are specific to the catabolism of glucose, the reactions of the citric acid cycle serve to degrade pyruvic acid or acetyl CoA derived from the breakdown of a variety of different food sources including proteins and fatty acids. A second difference between the two sections lies in the degree to which they depend on the supply of molecular oxygen. Thus, oxygen is essential for the functioning of the citric acid cycle, whereas the process of glycolysis can continue in its absence. Under such anaerobic conditions the pyruvic acid is not transformed to acetyl CoA but instead it is converted by a branch pathway to a more reduced end product such as ethanol or lactic acid. The rationale for this digression from the normal pathway will be explained later. Finally it is interesting to note that the division of the pathway is reflected in the organization of the cell. Thus all the enzymes which operate from pyruvate onwards are fixed to the mitochondrial membrane and thus operate in close association with the electron transport system, whereas the enzymes of glycolysis are not localized in this special compartment. The two sections will be treated separately in the following account.

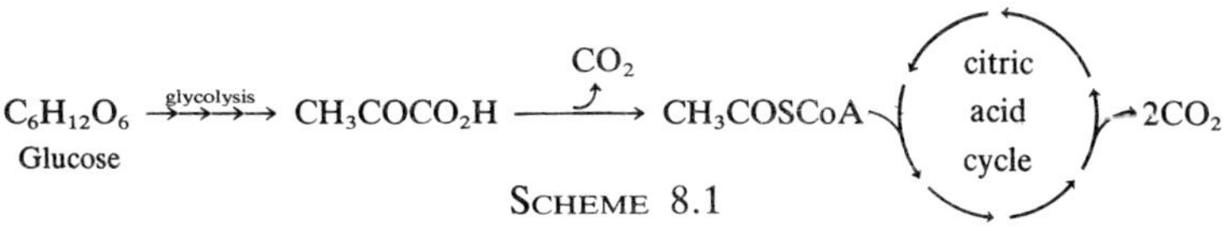

$$C_6H_{12}O_6 \xrightarrow{\text{glycolysis}} CH_3COCO_2H \xrightarrow{CO_2} CH_3COSCoA \xrightarrow{\text{citric acid cycle}} 2CO_2$$

Glucose

SCHEME 8.1

The pathway of glycolysis

A step by step commentary on this pathway, which leads to the conversion of a molecule of glucose to two of pyruvate is shown in Scheme 8.2.

Energetics

Considering first the energy balance in terms of ATP production, we can see that ATP is consumed in steps (1) and (3), but it is generated in steps (7) and (9). Since two C_3 units are generated in step (4), there is a net gain of two units of ATP for each molecule of glucose consumed. In addition NADH is generated in step (6), and under aerobic conditions this will be recycled in the electron transport system to furnish more ATP (6 units per mole of glucose).

However, this latter course is not open to an organism which is growing under anaerobic conditions. In this situation the production of NADH is potentially an embarrassment rather than an asset because it is necessary to find a way of reoxidizing the coenzyme that does not require molecular oxygen. In the fermentation of glucose by yeast this end is achieved by carrying out a non-oxidative decarboxylation of the pyruvic acid produced by glycolysis. The resultant acetaldehyde can then accept hydrogen from the NADH to form ethanol as in Scheme 8.3. No further energy is harnessed as a result of this step and its sole purpose is to recycle NADH to NAD^+ so that step (7) can operate on a continuous basis. The net effect of this mode of glycolysis is shown in Scheme 8.4.

SCHEME 8.2. The steps of glycolysis

$$HOH_2C-\underset{\underset{OH}{|}}{\overset{\overset{H}{|}}{C}}-\underset{\underset{OH}{|}}{\overset{\overset{H}{|}}{C}}-\underset{\underset{OH}{|}}{\overset{\overset{H}{|}}{C}}-\underset{\underset{OH}{|}}{\overset{\overset{H}{|}}{C}}-CHO$$

Glucose

(1) ⟋ ATP
(1) ⟍ ADP

(1) An example of phosphate ester formation driven by cleavage of ATP. This process releases free energy and so will help to start the flow of material in the desired direction. It is in effect a pumping stage on the metabolic pipeline.

$$\text{℗}OH_2C-\underset{\underset{OH}{|}}{\overset{\overset{H}{|}}{C}}-\underset{\underset{OH}{|}}{\overset{\overset{H}{|}}{C}}-\underset{\underset{OH}{|}}{\overset{\overset{H}{|}}{C}}-\underset{\underset{OH}{|}}{\overset{\overset{H}{|}}{C}}-CHO$$

Glucose-6-phosphate

(2)

(2) This type of isomerization in which an α-hydroxy aldehyde is interconverted with the corresponding α-hydroxy ketone is a common reaction in metabolism. The mechanism probably involves the common enol as will be explained later. In isolation this reaction is an evenly balanced equilibrium.

$$\text{℗}OH_2C-\underset{\underset{HO}{|}}{\overset{\overset{H}{|}}{C}}-\underset{\underset{OH}{|}}{\overset{\overset{H}{|}}{C}}-\underset{\underset{OH}{|}}{\overset{\overset{H}{|}}{C}}-\underset{\underset{O}{\|}}{C}-CH_2OH$$

Fructose-6-phosphate

(3) ⟋ ATP
(3) ⟍ ADP

(3) Another example of phosphate ester formation. This reaction will liberate free energy and so will effect the removal of fructose-6-phosphate formed in the previous step (i.e. it is another pumping stage).

$$\text{℗}OH_2C-\underset{\underset{OH}{|}}{\overset{\overset{H}{|}}{C}}-\underset{\underset{OH}{|}}{\overset{\overset{H}{|}}{C}}-\underset{\underset{OH}{|}}{\overset{\overset{H}{|}}{C}}-\underset{\underset{O}{\|}}{\overset{\overset{H}{|}}{C}}-CH_2O\text{℗}$$

Fructose-1,6-diphosphate

(4)

(4) The central carbon–carbon bond is cleaved in a process analogous to a reverse aldol condensation. The mechanism will be discussed later.

SCHEME 8.2. (Continued)

$$\underset{\text{3-Phosphoglyceraldehyde}}{\overset{H}{\underset{|}{\underset{OH}{\text{POH}_2\text{C}-\overset{|}{\underset{|}{\text{C}}}-\text{CHO}}}}} + \underset{\text{Dihydroxyacetone phosphate}}{\overset{}{\text{HOH}_2\text{C}-\overset{O}{\underset{||}{\text{C}}}-\text{CH}_2\text{OP}}}$$

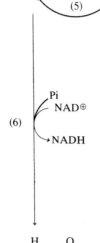

(5) The two products of step (4), a hydroxy aldehyde and a hydroxy ketone, are interconverted in a process related to step (2).

(6) The next enzyme operates on 3-phosphoglyceraldehyde which is removed as a result from the equilibria in steps (4) and (5). The aldehyde function is oxidized to the carboxylate level but the product is released at this stage as the acyl phosphate rather than the free carboxylic acid. This reaction is therefore an example of how oxidative phosphorylation can occur outside the electron transport system. The mechanism will be discussed later.

$$\underset{\text{1,3-Diphosphoglycerate}}{\overset{H}{\underset{|}{\underset{OH}{\text{POH}_2\text{C}-\overset{|}{\underset{|}{\text{C}}}-\overset{O}{\underset{OP}{\text{C}}}}}}}$$

(7) Cleavage of the acyl phosphate is coupled to ATP formation. Thus some of the energy liberated by the oxidation of the aldehyde is harnessed for the production of ATP and, taken together, steps (6) and (7) comprise a key process from the energetic point of view.

$$\underset{\text{3-Phosphoglycerate}}{\overset{H}{\underset{|}{\underset{OH}{\text{POH}_2\text{C}-\overset{|}{\underset{|}{\text{C}}}-\overset{O}{\underset{OH}{\text{C}}}}}}}$$

(8) The transfer of a phosphate from one alcoholic hydroxyl to another involves no great free-energy change but it sets the stage for the next key step.

(8)

Scheme 8.2. (Continued)

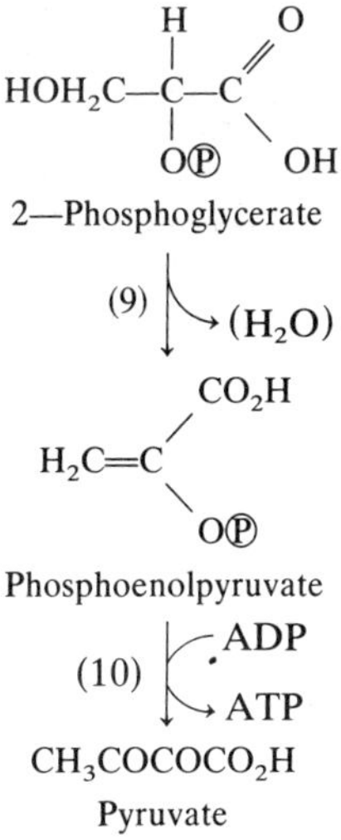

H   O
| //
HOH$_2$C—C—C
| \
O$\textcircled{P}$ OH

2—Phosphoglycerate

(9) $\big\downarrow$ (H$_2$O)

CO$_2$H
/
H$_2$C=C
\
O$\textcircled{P}$

Phosphoenolpyruvate

(10) $\big\{$ — ADP
     $\big\downarrow$ ATP

CH$_3$COCOCO$_2$H
Pyruvate

(9) and (10) As a result of these steps a further unit of ATP is generated. The underlying rationale of the process was discussed under oxidative phosphorylation in the last chapter and therefore no further comment is needed here, apart from noting that even though ATP is generated in step (10) there is still a considerable free-energy release and so this reaction will help to draw material forward from the previous step. In other words it serves as a 'waterfall' on the metabolic pipeline.

Note that no overall oxidation has taken place even though two molecules of carbon dioxide are generated. In fact the pathway brings about no more than a redistribution of the atoms of glucose into a more stable molecular arrangement and it can be calculated that the resultant yield of free energy is approximately 250 kJ mol^{-1}. Of this amount about 60 kJ mol^{-1} can be considered to be harnessed as a consequence of the net production of two moles of ATP, so the overall efficiency of the process is of the order of 25 per cent. However, it should be stressed that this measure of the efficiency represents no more than a notional value because it is calculated on the basis of free-energy data measured under standard conditions of concentration. In practice the reactions of metabolism take place under conditions more dilute so the true figure for the efficiency of the process could be markedly different.

The remaining free energy is dissipated in the form of heat but, of course, this loss is not completely wasteful. All the reactions of the pathway are potentially reversible and so some free energy must be sacrificed in this way if there is to be a decisive flow of materials in the required direction. This will ensure in turn that the concentration of ATP is maintained at a high level with respect to that of ADP. Reactions

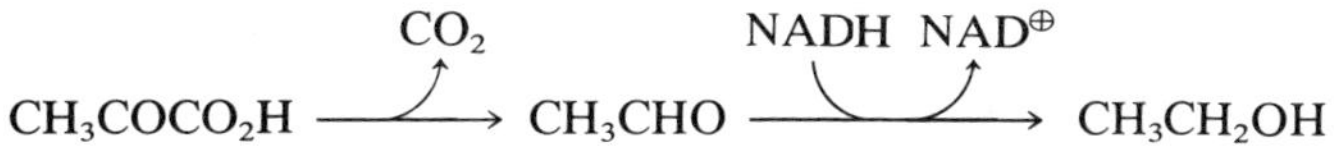

CH$_3$COCO$_2$H $\xrightarrow{\quad CO_2 \quad}$ CH$_3$CHO $\xrightarrow{\quad NADH \quad NAD^{\oplus} \quad}$ CH$_3$CH$_2$OH

Scheme 8.3

$$C_6H_{12}O_6 \longrightarrow 2CH_3CH_2OH + 2CO_2$$

SCHEME 8.4

(1), (3), (6), (7) and (10) have already been identified as steps which dissipate free energy, and, as a result, pull the overall process in the desired direction. Finally the diffusion of one of the end-products, carbon dioxide, away from the system will also help to achieve this end.

We have already seen that under normal aerobic conditions the pyruvate is subjected to oxidative decarboxylation to yield acetyl CoA which then enters the citric acid cycle. This type of transformation (involving thiamine, lipoic acid, a flavoprotein and NAD^+) was discussed at length in Chapter 5 and so no further comment is required apart from the reminder that, although NAD^+ is the immediate oxidant, the ultimate source of oxidizing power is provided by molecular oxygen acting through the agency of the electron transport system.

The rate of glucose catabolism is regulated primarily to meet the demand for ATP, and under normal conditions the enzymes of the citric acid cycle can cope adequately with the material produced by glycolysis so that there is no substantial build up of intermediates such as pyruvic acid or acetyl CoA. However, the citric acid cycle, which is indirectly responsible for the generation of a large proportion of the ATP, requires oxygen for its operation and as a result its maximum rate of operation is limited by the availability of molecular oxygen. Normally this presents no problem but under conditions of oxygen deficiency, such as can occur in the muscles of a mammal when working under stress, the throughput of the citric acid cycle may be severely limited by this factor. To some extent this shortfall in ATP production can be compensated by an increase in the rate of glycolysis but this can occur on a continuing basis only as long as there is an alternative to the electron transport system for reoxidizing the NADH generated in step (6). Fortunately, the pyruvic acid, which is generated at the same rate, provides a convenient solution to this problem by accepting hydrogen from the nicotinamide coenzyme to form lactic acid as in Scheme 8.5. This ploy allows the muscle cells to maintain ATP production at a higher rate than would otherwise be possible and no doubt many an animal has had cause to be thankful for the device when striving desperately to escape the jaws of a hungry predator.

The production of lactic acid in this way is in effect a variant of anaerobic glycolysis and in that sense the process is closely related to the

$$CH_3COCO_2H \xrightarrow{\quad NADH \quad NAD^{\oplus} \quad} CH_3CHOHCO_2H$$

SCHEME 8.5

fermentation of glucose to ethanol by yeast. However the lactic acid is not an end-product which is excreted but which accumulates in the muscle. Then, as soon as the oxygen supply is restored to an adequate level, the reaction shown in Scheme 8.5 can go into reverse and the resultant pyruvic acid can be metabolized via the citric acid cycle in the normal way.

Reaction mechanisms

It is not necessary to discuss each step of the pathway under this heading because several of them fall into one or other of the categories of reaction discussed at length in earlier chapters, and so will have received adequate coverage already.

Steps 2 and 5. The interconversion of an α-hydroxy ketone with the corresponding α-hydroxy aldehyde probably takes place via the inter-mediate enol as in Scheme 8.6. In principle at least two other mechanisms can be considered, involving migration of either the group R or the ringed hydrogen. However, in the biological reactions of this type which have been studied so far, the ringed hydrogen has been found to undergo exchange with protons of the medium as would be expected in the enolization process.

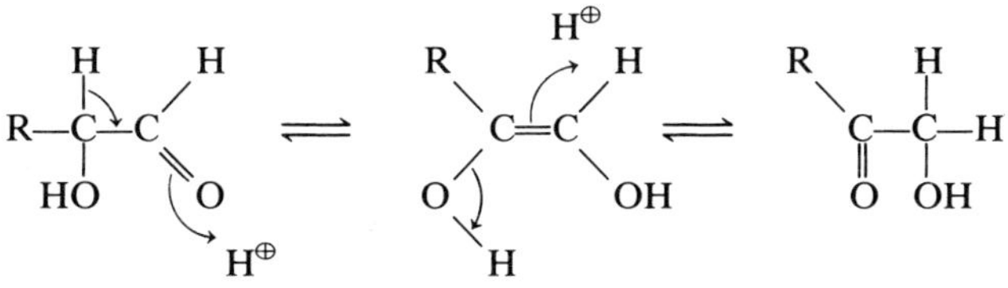

Scheme 8.6

Step (4): The aldolase reaction. This reaction takes place by cleavage of a β-hydroxy ketone grouping in a way that is reminiscent of a reverse aldol condensation. For that reason, the enzyme which catalyses the process has been given the name aldolase and the mechanism shown in Scheme 8.7 can be advanced. The key β-hydroxy ketone function is emphasized for clarity in the diagram.

Step (6): The oxidative phosphorylation. This key step, in which an aldehyde is oxidized to an acyl phosphate poses an interesting mechanistic problem. Scheme 8.8 shows a possible reaction sequence to account for the transformation. In the first step, nucleophilic addition of an enzyme-bound thiol group converts the aldehyde function to a thiohemiacetal [63], which is then oxidized to a thioester in a typical

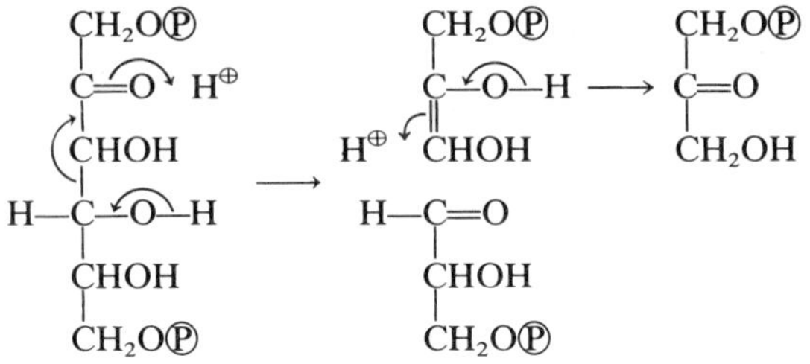

SCHEME 8.7

redox reaction with NAD$^+$. Subsequently, nucleophilic displacement of the thiol by inorganic phosphate leads in the standard way to an enzyme-free acyl phosphate.

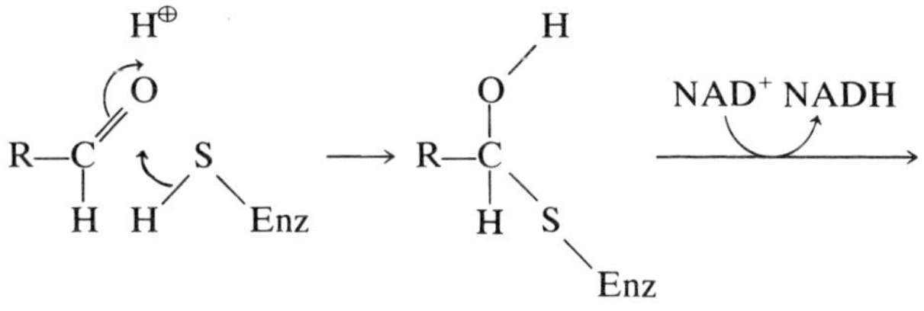

[63]

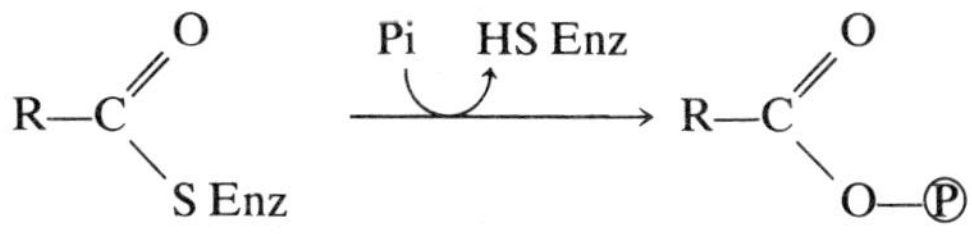

SCHEME 8.8

The citric acid cycle

The net effect of this sequence of reactions is to bring about the oxidation of an acetate group to two molecules of carbon dioxide. As its name implies this pathway is not linear but takes the form of a cycle of reactions. This feature complicates the following presentation because there is insufficient room on a page of this size to show the pathway in the form of a circle in the conventional way and to give at the same time a step by step commentary. Therefore the pathway will be drawn in linear form running down the side of the page in Scheme 8.9 and the reader will have to complete the cycle mentally by carrying the product of the final step back to the beginning.

SCHEME 8.9. The steps of the citric acid cycle

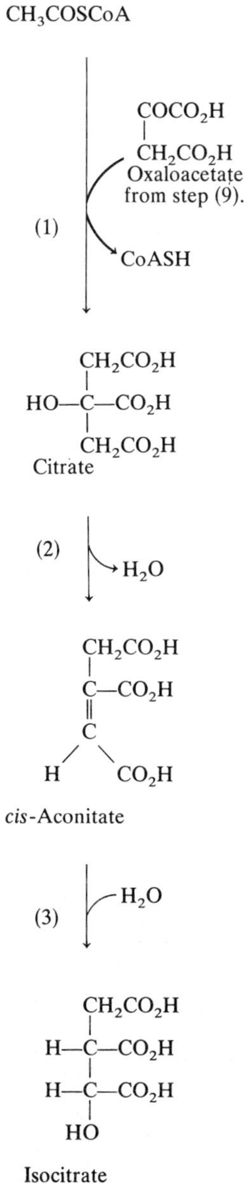

$CH_3COSCoA$

(1) The mechanism of this step probably involves a nucleophilic attack of the enolate of the thioester on the carbonyl group of oxalo-acetate as explained in Chapter 4. Note that this is a synthetic reaction in which a C_6-molecule is generated by combination of a C_2- with a C_4-molecule. The energetics of this step are particularly significant as will be explained later.

$COCO_2H$
$|$
CH_2CO_2H
Oxaloacetate
from step (9).

(1)

CoASH

CH_2CO_2H
$|$
$HO—C—CO_2H$
$|$
CH_2CO_2H
Citrate

(2)
H_2O

(2) and (3) The hydroxyl group is β to a carboxyl group and therefore it will undergo a ready elimination to give a $\alpha:\beta$-unsaturated acid. The reverse reaction will also take place readily by means of a nucleophilic addition to the β-carbon of the $\alpha:\beta$-unsaturated acid. However the double bond in *cis*-aconitic acid carries a carbonyl group at both ends and so the hydration can take place readily in the opposite sense to give isocitric acid (Step 3). In the absence of step (4) an equilibrium would be set up between citric and isocitric acids.

CH_2CO_2H
$|$
$C—CO_2H$
$\|$
C
$/$ $\backslash$
H CO_2H
cis-Aconitate

(3)
H_2O

CH_2CO_2H
$|$
$H—C—CO_2H$
$|$
$H—C—CO_2H$
$|$
HO

Isocitrate

SCHEME 8.9. (Continued)

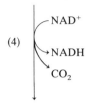

(4)   (4) This is the first redox reaction of the cycle. The mechanism will be discussed later.

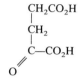

α-Ketoglutarate

(5)   (5) The mechanism of this oxidative decarboxylation, involving thiamine and lipoic acid as catalysts, was discussed at length in Chapter 5.

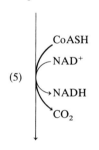

Succinyl CoA

(6)   (6) The thioester is cleaved with concommittant formation of a nucleoside triphosphate, GTP, from GDP and Pi. As explained in Chapter 5, this is equivalent to the generation of a unit of ATP.

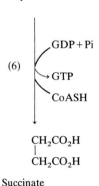

Succinate

SCHEME 8.9. (Continued)

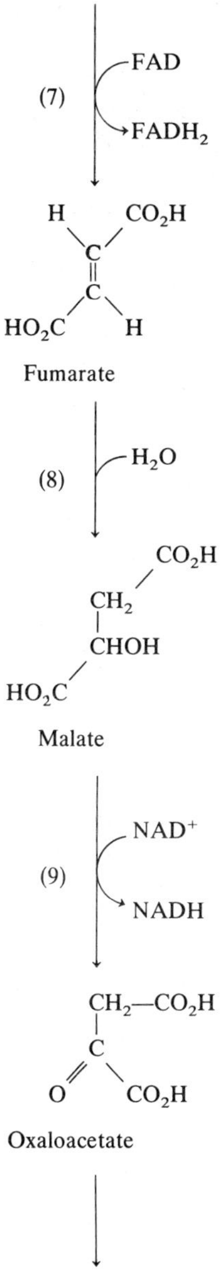

(7)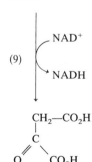

FAD

FADH$_2$

H   CO$_2$H

C

‖

C

HO$_2$C   H

Fumarate

(7) We are now left with a C$_4$ molecule and the aim of the subsequent steps is to oxidize one of the methylenes to a carbonyl group. The succinic acid is first dehydrogenated to fumaric acid by means of the electron transport system.

(8)

H$_2$O

CO$_2$H

CH$_2$

CHOH

HO$_2$C

Malate

(8) The double bond is then hydrated. This reaction is similar to the hydration of the double bond of *cis* -aconitic acid and will be assisted by the same factors.

(9)

NAD$^+$

NADH

CH$_2$—CO$_2$H

C

O   CO$_2$H

Oxaloacetate

(9) Finally, we see NADH carrying out a standard oxidation of a hydroxyl group to a carbonyl group. The cycle is now complete with a molecule of oxaloacetate ready to begin the next turn by combining with a fresh molecule of acetyl CoA.

To step (1).

Reaction mechanisms

The reactions taking place in steps (1), (5), (6), (7) and (9) have been covered in earlier chapters.

Steps (2), (3), *and* (8). As explained in the brief commentary these reactions are characteristic interconversions of β-hydroxy acids and $\alpha:\beta$-unsaturated acids. Possible mechanisms are shown in Scheme 8.10. In the dehydration process the carbonyl group assists in the removal of a proton from the α-carbon; in the reverse reaction it serves as an electron sink to assist in the nucleophilic addition of a hydroxide ion.

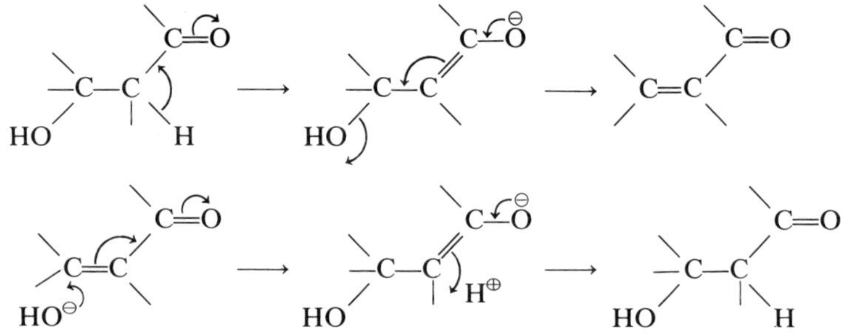

SCHEME 8.10

Step 4. A possible sequence of reactions for this transformation is given in Scheme 8.11. The first step is brought about by NAD^+ in a standard redox reaction. As a result, the central carboxyl function is placed β with respect to a ketonic carbonyl group and so it would be expected to undergo the required decarboxylation with ease. However, it has not been firmly established that the ketoacid is an obligatory intermediate in this reaction.

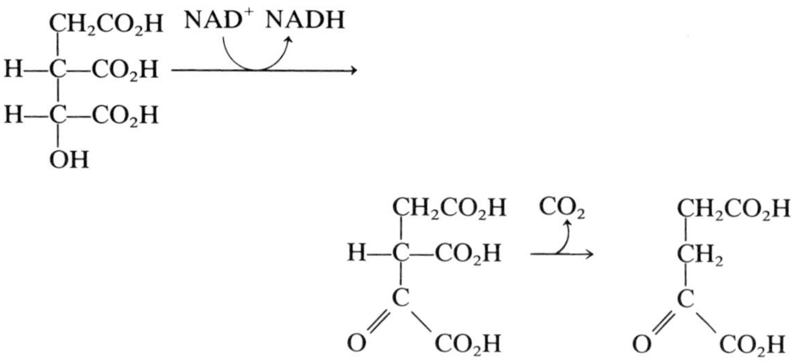

SCHEME 8.11

Energetics

The first step is particularly interesting in that the condensation of acetyl CoA and oxaloacetate leads to free citric acid rather than the corresponding coenzyme A ester, even though there is no absolute requirement on mechanistic grounds for the thioester group to be cleaved as a consequence of the condensation process. It might be thought therefore that this step of the pathway could be made more efficient from the point of view of bioenergetics by the evolution of two new enzymes. The first would condense oxaloacetate and acetyl CoA to form the coenzyme A ester of citric acid rather than the free acid; the second would then cleave the thioester to the free acid in a process coupled to the generation of ATP. However, this is the key stage at which fresh material is drawn into the cycle and the existing process has the advantage that by dissipating free energy, it serves as a 'waterfall' directing material from glycolysis into the citric acid cycle.

The next 'waterfall' comes in step (4) where isocitrate is oxidized to α-ketoglutarate, ultimately at the expense of molecular oxygen. Even though three units of ATP are generated in the electron transport system as a consequence of this transformation sufficient free energy is liberated to make the reaction essentially irreversible. This step has the effect of siphoning isocitrate from the equilibration with citrate and so ensures that steps (2) and (3) work in the required direction. The same considerations apply in the case of steps (7) and (9), each of which help to pull the previous step forward.

At this stage, it is interesting to take stock of the yield of ATP resulting from the oxidation of glucose to carbon dioxide and water. In all, 38 units of ATP are generated for each molecule of glucose consumed. Twelve units of this total are generated as a consequence of the glycolytic section of the pathway, which leaves 24 units to be generated in the citric acid cycle (12 units per turn). Of the latter, three units result from each of the steps (4), (5), and (9), two units are produced in step (7) and one as a consequence of step (6). It is also interesting to note that most of the ATP (34 units) is generated in the electron transport system and only four units result directly from the reactions of the pathway. These figures bring home the paramount importance of the system for the production of ATP in aerobic metabolism.

The strategy of glucose catabolism

When presented with a synthetic or degradative scheme, the organic chemist customarily looks for an underlying strategy and it is interesting to consider the pathway of glucose catabolism from this standpoint.

The section from glucose to acetyl CoA is essentially linear and has a straightforward strategy: the C_6 chain of glucose is cleaved to two C_3

units and the funtionality of each of these is modified in turn to produce two molecules of pyruvic acid; these are then cleaved to generate two acetyl units.

So far relatively little net oxidation has taken place and the main burden in this respect is borne by the reactions of the citric acid cycle. The strategy of this cyclic section of the pathway is less straightforward. Remarkably for a degradative scheme, the first step of the cycle is a synthetic process in which a C_4 molecule (oxaloacetate) is combined with a C_2 unit (an acetyl residue) to generate a C_6 molecule (citrate). This is then degraded over the next five steps to a C_4 molecule (succinic acid) plus two molecules of carbon dioxide. The subsequent steps bring about the oxidation of succinate to oxaloacetate without change in the carbon skeleton.

In a sense, therefore, the role of the C_4 unit is to act as carrier of the acetyl unit through the oxidation steps of the pathway. However, it should be explained that this simple analysis ignores a hidden complexity of the pathway revealed by tracer studies. Thus the two carbon atoms of a particular acetyl unit are not, as might be expected, liberated in the first turn of the cycle following their introduction but they emerge in a subsequent turn of the cycle. This phenomenon has its roots in the elements of symmetry present in the molecules of citric acid and succinic acid. It is of vital concern in tracer experiments because it leads to scrambling of the carbon labels but it is not important in the context of the present discussion and so it will not be discussed in detail.

Anaplerotic pathways

The pathway of glucose catabolism is of central importance by virtue of the contribution it makes to the energetics of living systems, but we should recognize that it makes a no less vital contribution in another sense, by providing many of the starting materials used by the biosynthetic pathways. Therefore, before closing this account, we shall survey briefly this alternative function of the pathway and in doing so we shall discover that a cyclic pathway presents a special problem in this sphere.

Many of the compounds produced as intermediates in the catabolism of glucose are employed as building blocks by the pathways of biosynthesis. For example, phosphoenolpyruvate and pyruvate are used in the synthesis of the amino acids phenylalanine and alanine respectively; acetyl CoA has been mentioned earlier as the precursor of the fatty acids; and moving on to the citric acid cycle we find that succinyl CoA can serve as a porphyrin precursor and α-ketoglutarate can be used in the production of glutamic acid.

In the case of a linear pathway such as that of glycolysis, the withdrawal of material from the pool of one of the intermediates can easily be compensated by an increase in the rate of the previous steps, so that the overall rate of the principal process need not be affected. However, when material is withdrawn from a cyclic pathway a special problem arises because the deficiency cannot be made good in the same straightforward manner.

Consider, for example, what would happen if succinyl CoA were to be withdrawn from the pool of intermediates available to the citric acid cycle in the absence of the compensating device to be discussed below: less oxaloacetate would be produced, and that would mean that the overall rate of operation would fall. In the extreme case the reactions would stop altogether when the pool of succinyl CoA was used up completely. In order to avoid this disastrous outcome any material removed from the pool of C_4 carrier metabolites at one point of the cycle must be replaced by feeding an equivalent amount of material into the cycle at another point.

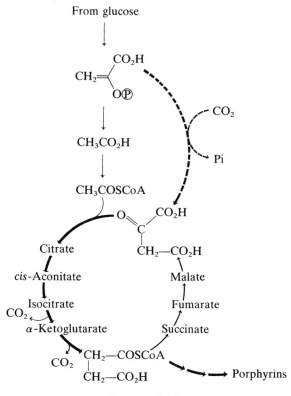

SCHEME 8.12

A process which fulfills this function (of maintaining the optimum level of a key metabolic pool) does not fit into either of the main categories of pathway (anabolic or catabolic) and so is placed in a special third category called the anaplerotic pathways. Scheme 8.12 shows a typical anaplerotic pathway (the dotted arrows) by which oxaloacetate can be generated directly from phosphoenol pyruvate, one of the intermediates of glycolysis. Thus whenever material is withdrawn from the pool of succinyl CoA for porphyrin biosynthesis this process can come into operation to supply an equivalent amount of replacement material in the form of oxaloacetate. The additional flow of material which would then take place is indicated in the scheme by heavy arrows.

As far as the normal pathway of glucose catabolism is concerned the anaplerotic pathway under consideration is in effect a by-pass which runs from phosphoenol pyruvate to oxaloacetate; this is why it is represented as such in the scheme and on the metabolic pathways map. There are many other anaplerotic pathways serving the citric acid cycle in this way and this fact accounts for many of the puzzling loops, by-passes, and cross-connections which appear on that part of the map.

9. Photosynthesis: the anabolism of glucose

No treatment of metabolism would be complete without at least a brief account of photosynthesis. As explained in Chapter 1, this amazing process converts the energy of sunlight into chemical energy and it can be justifiably regarded as the mainspring of the living world.

Since the radiant energy is used to bring about what amounts to a reversal of glucose catabolism, glucose and oxygen are produced from carbon dioxide and water (at least this is what happens in green plants, the only type of organism we shall consider), the logical place to deal with the topic is in this chapter, while the treatment of the catabolic pathway is still fresh. As we shall see, the latter process provides a useful basis for comparison when we come to analyse some aspects of photosynthesis.

Organization of the photosynthetic apparatus

Photosynthesis takes place as the result of the cooperative efforts of two separate sets of reactions which are called the light reactions and the dark reactions to indicate the degree to which they depend on light. The light reactions are absolutely dependent on radiant energy: as soon as the source of light is removed they stop. Their function is to harness the energy of light so as to effect the overall chemical changes shown in Scheme 9.1: NADP$^+$ is reduced to NADPH (using water as a reducing agent). As an added bonus, ATP is generated from ADP and inorganic phosphate. Note that the redox reaction presented in this scheme is essentially the reverse of the overall change that takes place in the electron transport system; hence the absolute dependence of the process on the provision of a suitable form of energy from outside.

The title dark reactions is accorded to the metabolic pathways along which material flows from carbon dioxide to glucose. This biosynthesis requires a supply of both energy and (given the nature of the overall chemical change) reducing power. These two requirements are met by the coenzymes produced as a consequence of the light reactions and

$$2H_2O \qquad \qquad 2NADPH$$
$$4H^{\oplus} + O_2 \qquad 4e \qquad 2NADP^{\oplus} + 2H^{\oplus}$$

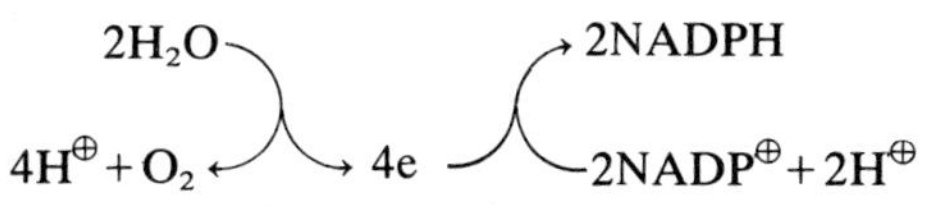

Scheme 9.1

radiant energy is not involved in any of the biosynthetic steps. Therefore the dark reactions will, as their name implies, continue to operate in the dark until the accumulated supply of NADPH and ATP is exhausted; given a suitable alternative source of these coenzymes, the reactions will operate indefinitely in the dark.

Hence the link between the light reactions and the dark reactions is a tenuous one (which recalls that which exists between the electron transport system and the pathway of glucose catabolism): the two systems are interconnected under normal circumstances by the associated coenzymes which shuttle back and forth between them, but each has the potential to operate independently of the other, given a suitable alternative means of recycling the attendant coenzymes. It is logical therefore, as well as convenient, to divide the subject along these lines and accordingly the light reactions and the dark reactions are treated in separate sections in the following account.

The light reactions: radiant energy into chemical energy

The enzymatic apparatus

In the cells of green plants the light reactions take place in special sub-cellular particles called the chloroplasts. These minute particles rival the mitochondria in complexity of structure and degree of organization. The effective operation of the light reactions is critically dependent on this structured environment and so the investigation of how they work is a challenging problem for the cell biologist as well as the chemist. In their general nature, the biological problems are closely related to those discussed earlier in connection with the electron transport system. It is not necessary, therefore, to go over similar ground here, and, accordingly, we will concentrate on the chemistry of the light reactions. It should be explained in addition that the following account gives a considerably simplified version of current theories, concentrating as it does on the general principles rather than the details, and also that many doubts and uncertainties are glossed over to avoid undue complication.

As explained earlier, the essential function of the light reactions is to carry out the reduction of $NADP^+$ to NADPH using water as reducing agent and the process boils down to the transfer of electrons (see Scheme 9.1). The way in which this transfer of electrons takes place is reminiscent of electron transport in mitochondria: in other words, the electrons travel through an electron transport chain passing from one component to the next in a series of interlocking redox reactions. In the photosynthetic apparatus, however, the electron flow takes place up an enormous energy hill. Therefore it is hopelessly unfavourable and we are faced with the question: how is this astonishing feat accomplished? The answer can be found in the special character of the electron transport chain, two stages of which are endowed with the remarkable ability to harness the energy of sunlight so as to drive an energetically unfavourable redox reaction. Photosynthesis hinges on these two stages. Therefore only those electron transfers which are directly associated with them will be discussed in detail below.

The components of the electron transport chain

First it is necessary to introduce the relevant components of the electron transport chain. One is a quinonoid cofactor of uncertain structure, which is believed to function by accepting one electron to form a semiquinone radical anion, as indicated in the partial structures [64] and [65] of Scheme 9.2. In order to save space in subsequent schemes the quinone will sometimes be represented by the symbol Q, and the radical anion by $[Q]^{\cdot-}$.

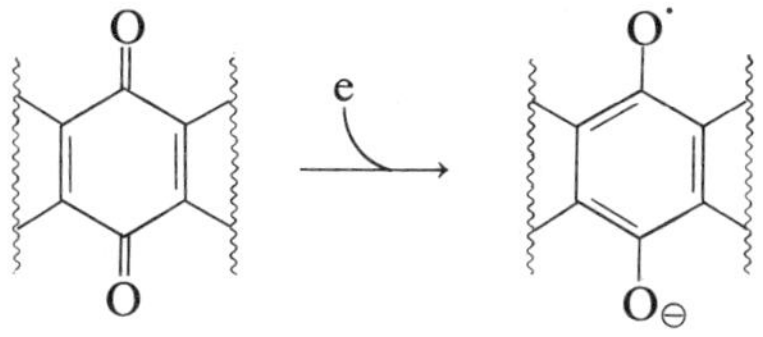

[64]   [65]

Scheme 9.2

A ferredoxin component also plays a part in one of the key stages. Diagram [66] shows a partial structure proposed for the active site of a typical ferredoxin (Cys indicates a cysteine residue); the rest of the molecule is protein. This astonishingly complex array of iron and sulphur residues seems to be characteristic of the ferredoxin family. The iron participates in the redox reactions by cycling between the Fe^{II} and Fe^{III} states and it is probable that its exceptionally high reducing potential ($E_0 = -0.4$ V) is largely determined by this unusual environment.

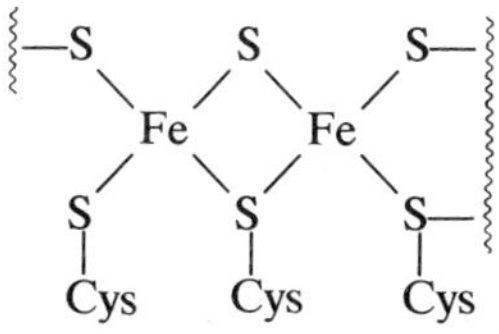

[66]

We now come to the prime mover of the photosynthetic apparatus, chlorophyll, the familiar green pigment of plants. The structure of a typical member of the chlorophyll family is shown [67]; other members

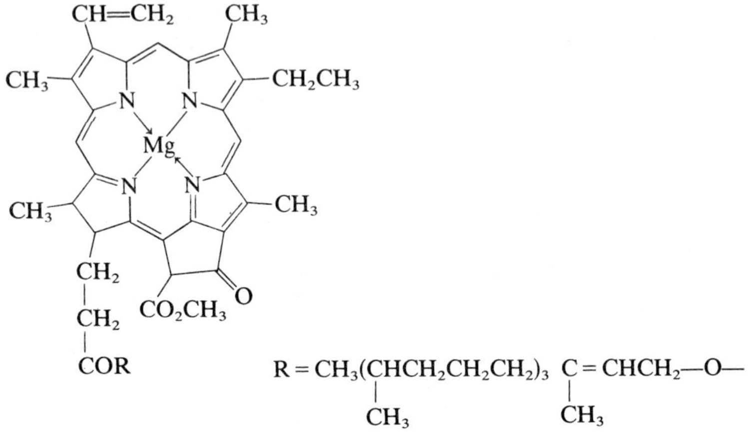
CH=CH2
CH3
CH3
CH2CH3
N
N
Mg
N
N
CH3
CH3
CH2
CH2
CO2CH3
O
COR
R = CH3(CHCH2CH2CH2)3 C = CHCH2—O—
CH3
CH3

[67] Chlorophyll a

of the family show minor variations in the structure of the side-chains which need not concern us here, since the seat of the photosynthetic ability of the chlorophyll structure lies in the system of conjugated π-bonds in the nucleus. This chromophore absorbs light in the visible region (and so gives rise to the green colour of the pigment). As usual the molecule is converted to an excited state when it absorbs light. Under normal conditions the excess energy of the excited state is dissipated into the environment but in the ordered environment of the photosynthetic apparatus the transformation shown in Scheme 9.3 can take place instead: the excited molecule, Chl*, donates an electron to a neighbouring acceptor (not specified here, but it will be the next component of the chain), and is converted as a result to a radical cation, $[Chl]^{+\cdot}$. The latter is a powerful oxidizing agent and in a subsequent step it abstracts an electron from a neighbouring donor (the preceding component) to revert to the ground state. The photoexcitation step is indicated in the scheme by a dotted line to distinguish it from the electron transfer steps.

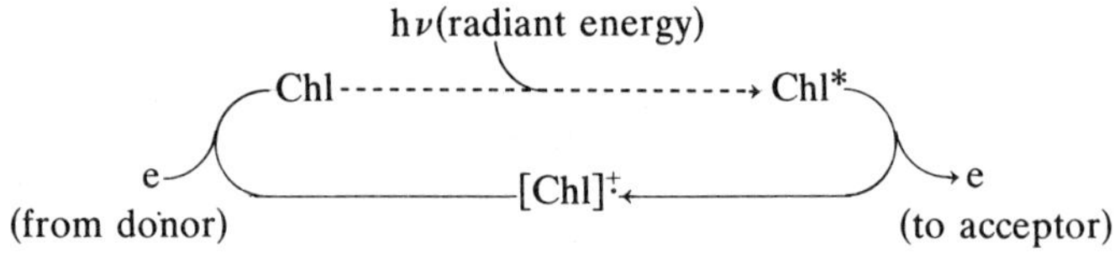
hν(radiant energy)
Chl
Chl*
e
(from donor)
[Chl]+·
e
(to acceptor)

Scheme 9.3

The electron donated by the chlorophyll is almost certainly provided by the extended.π-system (rather than, say, the central metal atom) and on that basis alone this is an unusual type of redox reaction. The energetics, however, are the really significant feature of the process for they hold the key to the conversion of sunlight energy into chemical energy. Thus a normal unexcited chlorophyll molecule does not have sufficient thermodynamic potential (in the reducing sense) to donate an electron to the neighbouring acceptor, but it becomes sufficiently energy rich to do so, as a consequence of photoexcitation. In a sense therefore, the energy absorbed from the light is used to 'pump' the electron up the energy hill leading from chlorophyll to the next component of the electron transport chain. In effect, light energy is converted to chemical energy and the initial objective of the photosynthetic apparatus is achieved.

The sequence of operations in the electron transport chain

We are now ready to examine the constitution of the electron transport chain, though, as explained earlier, only the components associated with the photoactive stages will be considered. The sequence in which they operate is shown in Scheme 9.4. Note that two chlorophylls, Chl$_I$

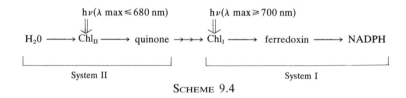

$$H_2O \longrightarrow Chl_{II} \longrightarrow quinone \rightarrow\rightarrow\rightarrow Chl_I \longrightarrow ferredoxin \longrightarrow NADPH$$

SCHEME 9.4

and Chl$_{II}$, are involved. These are associated with the two photoactive stages which are designated system I and system II as indicated. The chlorophylls differ somewhat in the wavelength of light which they can use most efficiently and also (as we shall see below) in their redox potentials. The disparity in the latter property is particularly important for photosynthesis; presumably it arises because the two chlorophyll components of the chain operate in markedly different environments.

Oxygen evolution takes place in system II at the start of the chain and Scheme 9.5 shows how the electrons are transferred as far as the quinone component. First, the chlorophyll is excited by light to transfer an electron to the quinone. The resulting radical cation, [Chl]$^{\ddot{+}}$, is an extremely powerful oxidizing agent and therefore has the ability to abstract an electron from water. Note that (a) a total of four electrons have to be transferred in this way for each molecule of oxygen liberated;

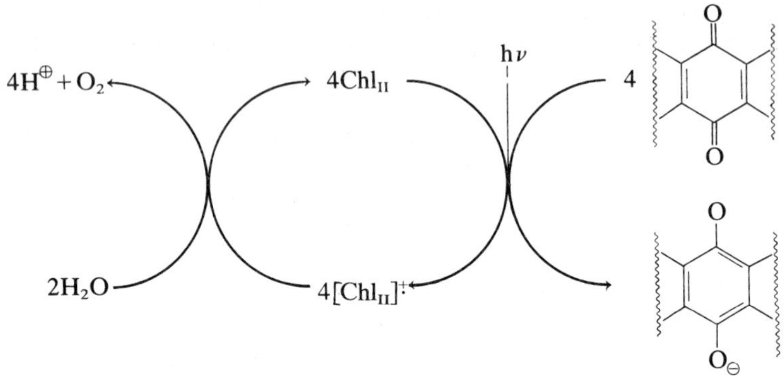

SCHEME 9.5

(b) protons are the other by-product of the oxidation of water; and (c) for every electron transferred a molecule of radical anion is produced on the right. Obviously, the latter has to be recycled to quinone if the reaction is to operate as a continuous basis. We shall return to this point below.

The reactions of system I are shown in Scheme 9.6. First, the electron is driven by photoexcitation to a neighbouring acceptor, this time a ferredoxin. The reduced form of the latter then reduces $NADP^+$ to the dihydro form. Once again several points should be noted: (a) for every molecule of NADPH produced two electrons undergo transfer (whether these are transferred to the nicotinamide simultaneously from two adjacent ferredoxins, or successively from one such component is not known); (b) the hydrogen added to the nicotinamide is derived from the protons of water (whether it is added as H^+, H^- or $H^{\cdot}$ remains to be discovered); (c) the chlorophyll is left in the form of a radical cation and needs to be supplied with electrons to complete its cycle. This is where the centre section of the chain (see Scheme 9.4) comes into play. The radical anion produced by system II transfers its odd electron through this section (it consists of a series of cytochromes) to the radical cation

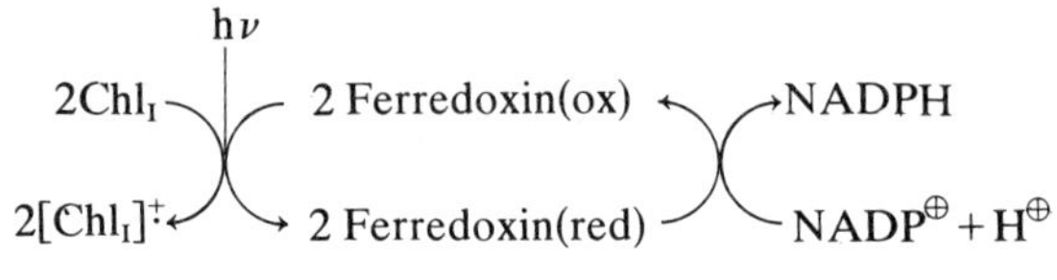

SCHEME 9.6

derived from system I. Hence we have now traced a complete pathway for electron transfer from water through to the nicotinamide coenzyme.

The energetics of the redox reactions

Our next task in this analysis of the light reactions is to analyse the energetics of the various electron transfer steps on the basis of the redox potentials of the various components. Remember that in the electron transport chain of the mitochondria these values become steadily more positive as one moves from one component to the next in the direction of electron flow. Hence each transfer is favourable and the electron flow takes place down an energy hill.

The sequence of redox potentials of the photosynthetic chain presents a markedly different picture and this is illustrated graphically in Scheme 9.7 where the components (each shown in the reduced form) run in sequence from left to right, the direction of electron flow. The position of each component is plotted against a vertical scale according to the value of its redox potential: the higher up a given component appears on the diagram, the greater its potential for donating an electron.

It is now clear that the electron travels up and down energy hills on its passage through the photosynthetic chain. The diagram should be largely

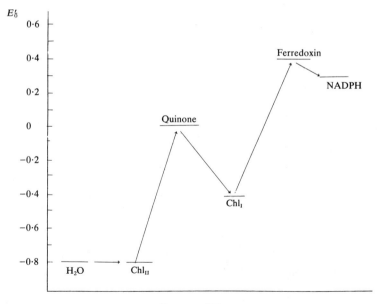

SCHEME 9.7

self-explanatory but in case they are missed the following points will be mentioned. First, the electron is pumped up an energy hill in two steps; otherwise the flow takes place downhill. Second, both photoactive steps pump the electron through roughly the same distance (0·8 V) and this is not sufficient to span the total energy gap between water and NADPH (~1·1 V). Therefore the two systems need to operate in collaboration and this is made possible by the disparity in the redox potentials of the two chlorophylls (the actual value for the chlorophyll of system II is not certain; it is placed where it is on the diagram to indicate that its radical cation will abstract an electron from water).

The third point to note is that in going from the quinone component to the chlorophyll of system II the electron runs down a sizeable energy hill and so energy is liberated. Nature, ever watchful for any opportunity to improve the efficiency of her metabolic machines, does not allow this energy to go to waste as heat; on the contrary, she has adapted this stage of the chain in the course of evolution so that the energy can be harnessed to generate ATP by oxidative phosphorylation of ADP. Hence the photosynthetic apparatus is revealed as an astonishingly ingenious device for converting light energy into chemical energy and its effectiveness in this respect is determined to a large extent by the finely tuned energetics of the sequence of redox reactions.

Finally, before leaving the subject of the light reactions, it should be explained, lest the reader feels they might have been overlooked, that virtually nothing is known about the electronic mechanisms of the various redox reactions. Moreover the problems are far too complex for speculation to be worthwhile here (though the nature of some of them has been hinted at earlier). Many research groups are active in this area and hopefully their efforts will soon supply the answers to the many questions which need to be resolved.

The dark reactions

In this section we shall be concerned with the various metabolic pathways which lead to the conversion of carbon dioxide to glucose. The overall material balance in the formation of a molecule of glucose is shown in Scheme 9.8. Note the heavy consumption of both NADPH and ATP, both of which are, of course, regenerated by the light reactions.

$$6CO_2 + \begin{cases} 12\,NADPH \\ + \\ 18\,ATP \\ + \\ 12\,H_3O^{\oplus} \end{cases} \longrightarrow C_6H_{12}O_6 + \begin{cases} 12\,NADP^{\oplus} \\ + \\ 18\,ADP \\ + \\ 18\,Pi \end{cases}$$

SCHEME 9.8

Though the overall preparative result of the biosynthesis amounts to a reversal of glucose catabolism, the dark reactions do not involve a step by step reversal of the catabolic pathways discussed in the last chapter. Instead a very different general strategy is followed in which material flows through a complex set of interlocking cyclic pathways. The wider strategy of this set of pathways will be considered more fully later. For the moment we shall concentrate on the much simpler task of analysing the central pathway of the set, which is the one that leads directly from carbon dioxide to glucose and carries the net flow of material out of the network biosynthetic pathways.

The central pathway

This pathway is shown in Scheme 9.9. Note that in addition to carbon dioxide a molecule of ribulose-1,5-diphosphate is consumed in step (1); we shall consider the source of this starting material later. The subsequent sequence of reactions is effectively a step by step reversal of the pathway by which glucose is degraded to 3-phosphoglycerate during the early stages of glycolysis [steps (1) to (7) of Scheme 8.2]. The mechanisms of these reactions have been covered adequately in Chapter 8 and so they will not be considered in detail here. Therefore, the main point of interest lies in the energetics of the reactions and in the following treatment we shall attempt to answer this question: what factors cause material to flow towards glucose on the anabolic pathway but away from glucose on the catabolic pathway?

SCHEME 9.9 The pathway from CO_2 to glucose.

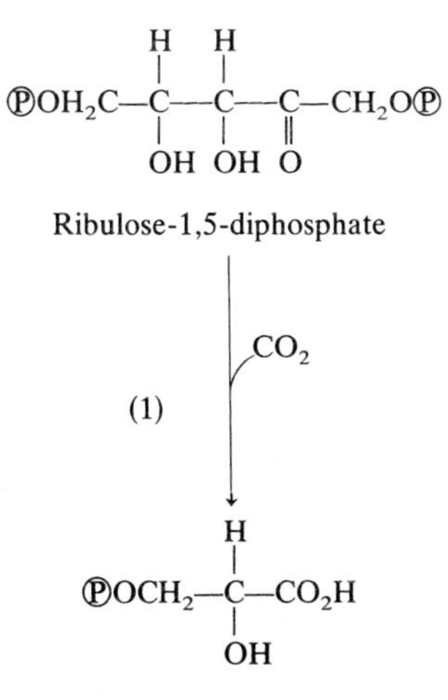

Ribulose-1,5-diphosphate

(1) This is the pivotal step of the biosynthesis at which CO_2 is assimilated. Note that two molecules of 3-phosphoglycerate will be produced.

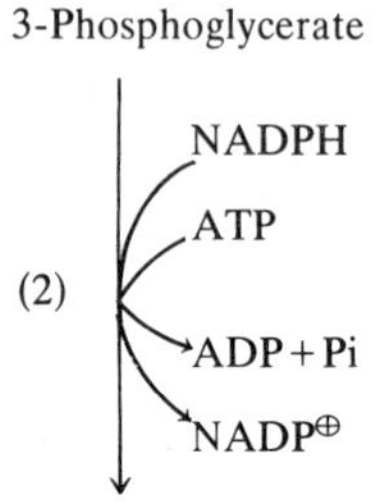

3-Phosphoglycerate

(2)

NADPH

ATP

ADP + Pi

NADP⊕

(2) This step corresponds to a reversal of steps (6) and (7) of the glycolysis pathway. Presumably therefore the mechanism involves initial formation of an energy-rich acyl phosphate. This (or an enzyme-bound thioester derived from it) would then be reduced by transfer of hydride from the nicotinamide coenzyme.

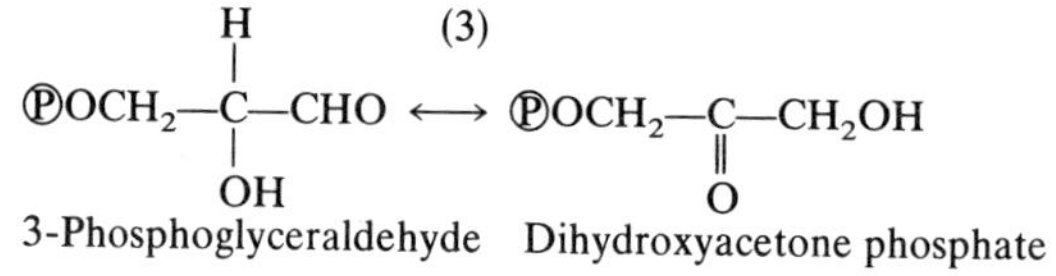

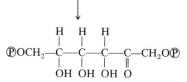

(3)

Ⓟ OCH₂—C—CHO ⟷ Ⓟ OCH₂—C—CH₂OH
   | ‖
   H OH   O

3-Phosphoglyceraldehyde   Dihydroxyacetone phosphate

(4)

(3) This interconversion presumably takes place via the common enol.

$$Ⓟ OCH_2—\underset{OH}{\overset{H}{C}}—\underset{OH}{\overset{H}{C}}—\underset{OH}{\overset{H}{C}}—\underset{O}{C}—CH_2OⓅ$$

Fructose-1,6-diphosphate

(4) An aldol condensation involving nucleophilic attack by the enol form of the ketone on the aldehyde (cf. step 4 of glycolysis).

(5)

Pi

(5) A simple hydrolysis of a phosphate ester. This is a key step for the energetics of the pathway as will be explained below.

$$Ⓟ OCH_2—\underset{OH}{\overset{H}{C}}—\underset{OH}{\overset{H}{C}}—\underset{OH}{\overset{H}{C}}—\underset{O}{C}—CH_2OH$$

Fructose-6-phosphate

(6)

(6) Interconversion via the common enol.

$$Ⓟ OH_2C—\underset{OH}{\overset{H}{C}}—\underset{OH}{\overset{H}{C}}—\underset{OH}{\overset{H}{C}}—\underset{OH}{\overset{H}{C}}—CHO$$

SCHEME 9.9 (Continued)

Glucose-6-phosphate

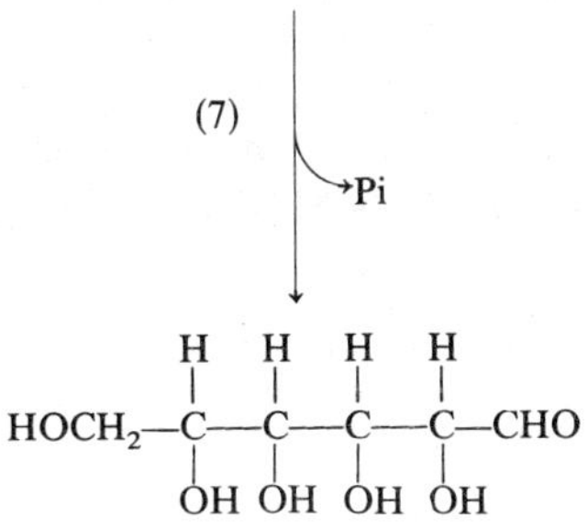

(7)

→Pi

(7) Another simple hydrolysis of a phosphate ester. Again the reaction is a key one for the energetics of the pathway.

$$\text{HOCH}_2-\overset{\overset{\displaystyle H}{|}}{\underset{\underset{\displaystyle OH}{|}}{C}}-\overset{\overset{\displaystyle H}{|}}{\underset{\underset{\displaystyle OH}{|}}{C}}-\overset{\overset{\displaystyle H}{|}}{\underset{\underset{\displaystyle OH}{|}}{C}}-\overset{\overset{\displaystyle H}{|}}{\underset{\underset{\displaystyle OH}{|}}{C}}-\text{CHO}$$

Glucose

Energetics. Since the first reaction of the pathway is novel it is desirable to consider its mechanism. The one proposed in Scheme 9.10 is based on analogy with the chemistry of β-keto acids and their derivatives. Thus, the first two stages of the scheme are equivalent to a reversal of the standard decarboxylation of β-keto acids and stages (iii) and (iv) involve a carbon-carbon cleavage, that is closely related to the typical cleavage of β-keto esters on treatment with base.

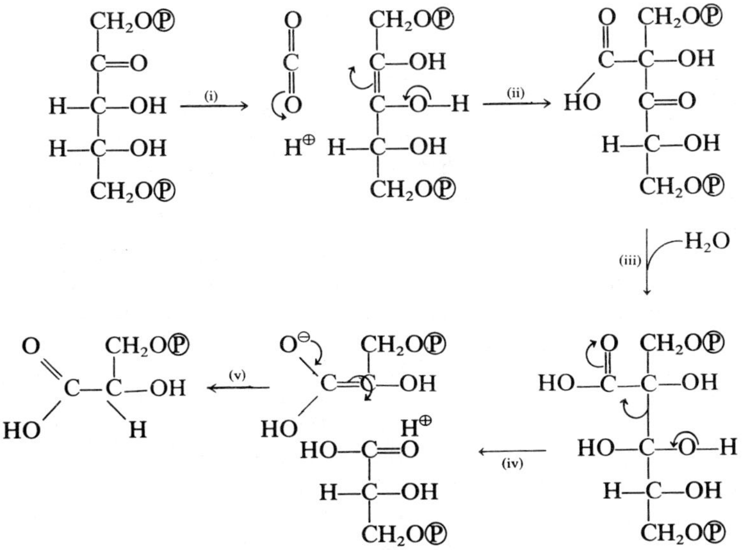

SCHEME 9.10

The energetics of this transformation deserve comment. Normally a carboxylation such as that which takes place in stages (i) and (ii) has an adverse equilibrium and would not be preparatively useful (this topic will be developed more fully in the next chapter). In this case, however, the carboxylation is coupled in the enzyme-mediated reaction to the subsequent cleavage of a carbon-carbon bond, and the favourable energetics of the latter process will help to compensate for the adverse character of the former.

The anabolic process: step (2) of Scheme 9.9:

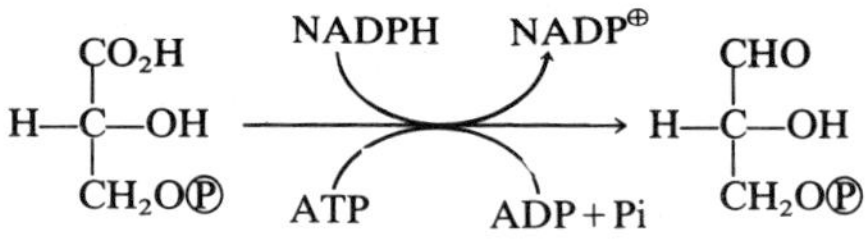

The catabolic process: steps (6) and (7) of Scheme 8.2:

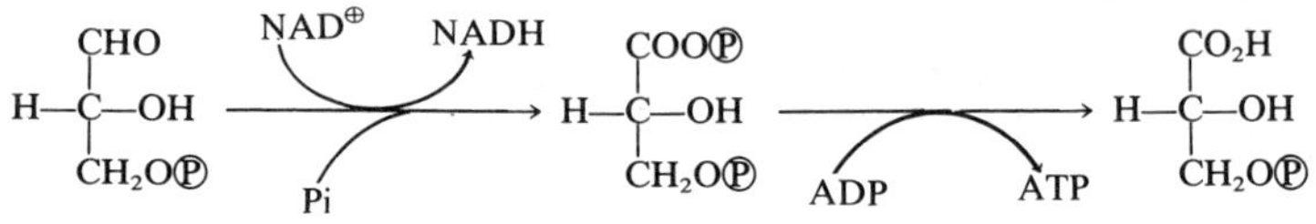

SCHEME 9.11

Step (2) of the metabolic pathway is also remarkable from the thermo-dynamic point of view, for it is equivalent to a direct reversal of two of the key steps of glycolysis. To help make this clear the two transformations are shown together in Scheme 9.11 (the fact that the catabolic process takes place in two steps is incidental to the following discussion). In the discussion of the energetics of the catabolic pathway (Chapter 8) it was argued that, even allowing for the generation of ATP, the overall transformation shown in Scheme 9.11 would release free energy, and that as a result the flow of material would run downhill at this stage in the direction of carboxylic acid formation. We are faced with a question therefore: what factor assists the uphill flow of material when the process operates in the reverse direction on the anabolic pathway? Or to put the question in more familiar terms: what aspect of the anabolic process causes the position of the notional equilibrium to be displaced in favour of the aldehyde?

The answer lies in the identity of the associated nicotinamide coenzyme. The catabolic process employs the couple $NAD^+/NADH$ as cofactor. Typically this coenzyme is maintained mainly in the oxidized form as a consequence of the oxidizing power of the electron transport system. It has, therefore, high potential for carrying out oxidations and accordingly the position of equilibrium in the metabolic redox reactions with which it is associated will be biased in favour of the oxidized product. Conversely the couple $NADP^+/NADPH$ is employed in the anabolic process. The pool of this coenzyme is maintained predominantly in the reduced form (by the operation of the light reactions of the photosynthetic apparatus, in the case under consideration), and as a result, the position of equilibrium in the anabolic reaction will be displaced in favour of the reduced product. Hence the notional point of equilibrium (and therefore the favourable direction of operation) of each of these conflicting metabolic transformations is determined by pressure from an external driving force (here the electron transport system or the light reactions of the photosynthetic apparatus) which acts indirectly through the pool of the associated nicotinamide coenzyme.

Steps (5) and (7) of the anabolic pathway also play a part in determining the net direction of flow. Each of these reactions involves a simple hydrolytic cleavage of a phosphate ester (i.e. the process is not coupled to the formation of ATP) and therefore free energy will be liberated when material flows in the required direction. The corresponding steps of the catabolic pathway must, therefore, be inherently unfavourable from the thermodynamic point of view, and in each case it is necessary to overcome this hurdle by coupling phosphate ester formation to the cleavage of ATP. We have seen this tactic in use on many occasions in earlier chapters, though it should be noted that the pathways under consideration here are hardly typical in the way they make use of it, for the pumping stations operate on the catabolic pipeline and not, as is usually the case, on the anabolic pipeline.

To sum up, therefore, we have identified two factors which determine that the direction of flow on the catabolic pathway is opposite to that on the anabolic pathway. First, certain key steps are coupled to ATP cleavage on one pathway but not on the other. Second, the two pathways differ in their choice of nicotinamide coenzyme for carrying out a key redox reaction, each selecting the cofactor appropriate to its aim. In contrast to the many references to the first tactic in earlier chapters, the second has only been briefly mentioned so far (in Chapter 6). Nevertheless, the latter working arrangement, which is based on the existence of two separate and independent pools of nicotinamide coenzymes, makes a vital contribution to the controlled working of every major area of metabolism and it will be necessary to refer to it on many occasions in subsequent chapters.

Finally, to keep the above discussion in perspective, it should be remembered that we have considered up to now only a small fraction of the reactions which participate in glucose biosynthesis. The transformations which take place in the rest of the biosynthetic network will also have an indirect influence on the direction of operation of the central pathway because they supply one of the starting materials (ribulose-1,5-diphosphate) and also remove material from the pools of certain intermediates (e.g. 3-phosphoglycerate). In spite of this omission the treatment given above is valid as far as it goes, and it provides a useful insight into the nature of the questions which need to be considered when comparing an anabolic pathway with the corresponding catabolic pathway.

The production of ribulose-1,5-diphosphate

The flow of material along the pathway from carbon dioxide to glucose only accounts for a small fraction of the total flow which is associated with glucose biosynthesis, for the central pathway can operate on a continuous basis only as long as it is provided with a continuous supply of its second starting material ribulose-1,5-diphosphate.

This is where the complex set of biosynthetic cycles mentioned earlier play their part. For every twelve C_3 molecules (i.e. 3-phosphoglycerate) produced in step (1) of the central pathway only two continue as far as glucose; the remaining ten are recycled to produce six molecules of the C_5 starting material.

The conversion of ten C_3 molecules into six C_5 molecules (all ribulose-1,5-diphosphate) clearly requires a complex reorganization. One of the pathways which contributes to this task is given in detail in Scheme 9.12. It starts with a C_6 compound, fructose-1,6-diphosphate (equivalent to two C_3 units), and a C_3 compound, 3-phosphoglyceraldehyde). These are siphoned off on a one to one basis from the respective intermediate pools on the central pathway.

As explained in the commentary the C_4 by-product of the first step is diverted so that it follows a different route to ribulose-1,5-diphosphate. It

SCHEME 9.12. A pathway leading to ribulose-1,5-diphosphate.

CHO
|
H—C—OH
|
CH$_2$O℗

Glyceraldehyd-
3-phosphate

CH$_2$OH
|
C=O
|
HO—C—H
|
H—C—OH
|
H—C—OH
|
CH$_2$O℗

Fructose-6-
phosphate

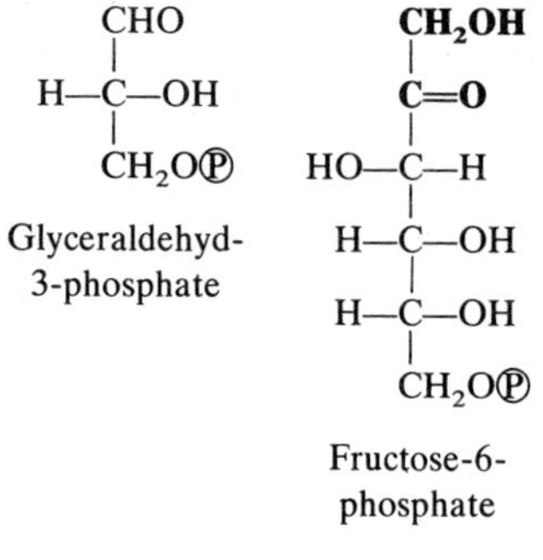

SCHEME 9.12 (Continued)

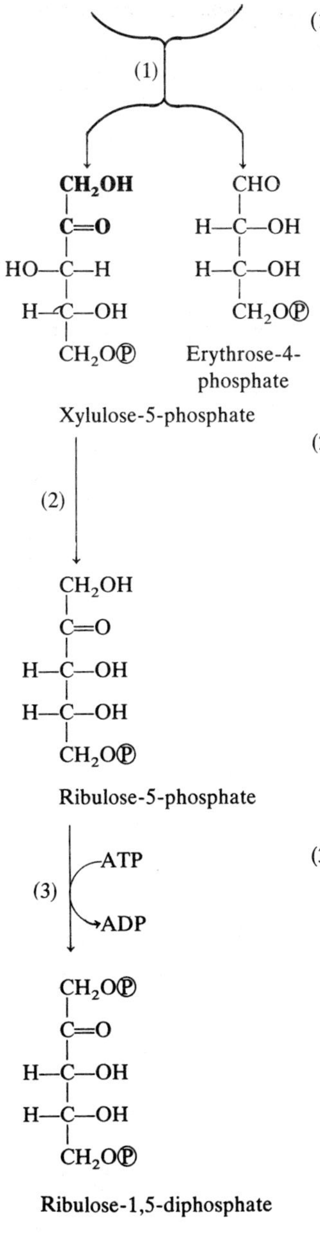

(1) This is the key step in which the carbon skeletons are reorganized by transfer of a C_2 unit (shown in heavy type) from the C_6 molecule to the C_3 molecule. The reaction is an example of transketolization mediated by the coenzyme thiamine pyrophosphate and its mechanism was discussed in Chapter 5. The erythrose-4-phosphate leaves the pathway at this point.

CH₂OH ... C=O ... HO—C—H ... H—C—OH ... CH₂OⓅ

Xylulose-5-phosphate

CHO ... H—C—OH ... H—C—OH ... CH₂OⓅ

Erythrose-4-phosphate

(2) The asymmetric centre at C-3 is epimerized presumably via enolization of the neighbouring carbonyl group.

CH₂OH ... C=O ... H—C—OH ... H—C—OH ... CH₂OⓅ

Ribulose-5-phosphate

(3) A standard phosphorylation. The cleavage of ATP will pump the flow of material in the required direction.

ATP → ADP

CH₂OⓅ ... C=O ... H—C—OH ... H—C—OH ... CH₂OⓅ

Ribulose-1,5-diphosphate

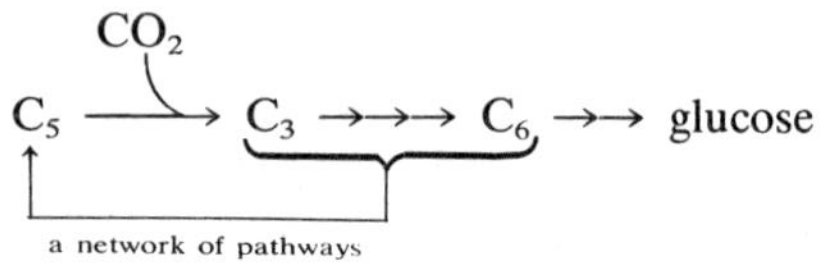

$$CO_2$$
$$C_5 \longrightarrow C_3 \rightarrow\rightarrow\rightarrow C_6 \rightarrow\rightarrow glucose$$

a network of pathways

SCHEME 9.13

is not necessary, however, to trace everyone of the network of pathways leading to this goal. The important point is the net direction of flow and the overall material balance which are shown in Scheme 9.13.

Material passes continuously in a clockwise direction through the cyclic pathways on the left and as a consequence carbon dioxide is assimilated into the pool of metabolites. The extra material which results is leaked steadily from the system along the central pathway described earlier. As long as the rate at which C_6 molecules are removed is maintained at one sixth of the rate of carbon dioxide assimilation, a steady state will obtain in which the total amount of material flowing round cyclic pathways remains constant. The overall result of this steady state was summarized at the outset in Scheme 9.8: for every six molecules of carbon dioxide incorporated, one of glucose is produced, and the supply of NADPH and ATP produced by the light reactions is put to good use.

10. Fatty acid metabolism

Structure and metabolic role

THE TERM fatty acid applies generally to all the long-chain fatty acids elaborated by living organisms. Within this class there is a considerable variety of structure and some representative examples are shown in Scheme 10.1.

$$CH_3(CH_2)_{14}CO_2H \qquad \text{Palmitic acid}$$

$$CH_3(CH_2)_{16}CO_2H \qquad \text{Stearic acid}$$

$$CH_3(CH_2)_7CH{=}CH(CH_2)_7CO_2N \qquad \text{Oleic acid}$$

$$CH_3(CH_2)_4CH{=}CHCH_2CH{=}CH(CH_2)_7CO_2H \qquad \text{Linoleic acid}$$

$$CH_3(CH_2)_5{-}\triangle{-}(CH_2)_9CO_2H \qquad \text{Lactobacillic acid}$$

$$CH_3CH_2\underset{\underset{CH_3}{|}}{CH}(CH_2)_{10}CO_2H \qquad \text{12-Methyltetradeceanoic acid}$$

SCHEME 10.1

Compounds of this type are involved in many different biological roles but the only one we need consider is their function in the sphere of energy storage.

We have already seen how carbohydrates such as glucose serve in this capacity and we shall find that fatty acids function in essentially the same way. Thus on total combustion they release a considerable amount of free energy and the living cell is able to carry out this process in a controlled way so that much of the energy can be harnessed for the production of ATP. Conversely fatty acids can be biosynthesized by a route which leads to the consumption of chemical energy and so they have the potential to act as an energy store, being synthesized when energy is available in excess of immediate requirements and degraded when it is in short supply.

It must be emphasized, however, that the fatty acids cannot be synthesized directly from carbon dioxide. Therefore they do not provide an independent alternative to photosynthesis and are best viewed as an accessory to carbohydrate metabolism, as illustrated in Scheme 10.2. Here we see glucose, produced by photosynthesis (or perhaps consumed as food), being degraded by glycolysis in the normal way to acetyl CoA which can then serve as the synthetic building block for fatty acid biosynthesis. Consequently, any temporary excess of glucose need not be

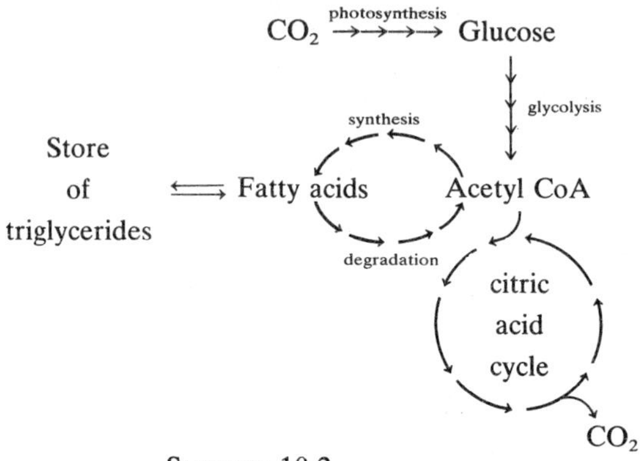

$$CO_2 \xrightarrow{\text{photosynthesis}} \text{Glucose}$$

SCHEME 10.2

stored as such or in the form of a carbohydrate polymer, but it may be converted instead to a fatty acid. Subsequently, when insufficient glucose is available to meet the demand for acetyl CoA, the deficiency can be made good by degrading material from the fatty acid store.

For reasons which will become clear when we discuss the pathways in detail, only straight-chain fatty acids having an even number of carbon atoms serve in this way and the most important are those with fourteen, sixteen, or eighteen carbons. The chain may be saturated or unsaturated. Of the structures shown in Scheme 10.1 the first four meet these criteria and all are involved in energy storage. As implied in Scheme 10.2, the fatty acid is stored not as the free acid but in the form of a triglyceride derivative, the corresponding triester of glycerol, with which it can be readily interconverted. Structure [68] shows the triglyceride derivative of stearic acid and compounds of this type form the bulk of the material stored in the fatty tissues of mammals.

At this stage it is reasonable to ask what benefit, if any, is gained from the practice of storing energy in the form of fats rather than carbohydrates. The answer to this question can be sought by comparing the structures of the two compounds. In contrast to glucose, and for that matter most other metabolites of the central pathways, the fatty acid structure is in an almost completely reduced state with a correspondingly low oxygen content, and, consequently, it provides a potentially more efficient means of energy storage on the basis of free-energy content per

$$CH_2-O-CO(CH_2)_{16}CH_3$$
$$CH-OCO(CH_2)_{16}CH_3$$
$$CH_2-O-CO(CH_2)_{16}CH_3$$

[68]

unit weight. Nevertheless both systems of storing energy are widely used by living organisms. Thus, while plants store their energy mainly in carbohydrate form, mammals use carbohydrates to a very small extent and rely instead on fatty acids for the major part of their requirements. This pattern accords well with the contrasting needs of the two types of organism. Mammals are mobile and speed of movement is a crucial factor governing the survival of the species and consequently, there is an urgent need to keep weight and bulk to a minimum. On the other hand, a typical plant remains rooted throughout its life to one place. Moreover its extensive aerial and underground parts provide ample room for storage of material. It follows that weight and bulk no longer represent a serious disadvantage and since there is no longer a powerful incentive to convert carbohydrates to fats it comes as no surprise to find that bulbs and tubers for instance are rich in carbohydrate but contain virtually no fat. Nevertheless plants do show an interesting change from their usual pattern of metabolism at the time of sexual reproduction, for the seeds of many species contain a high proportion of vegetable oils. These oils are the triglyceride derivatives of unsaturated fatty acids such as linoleic acid. As such they are biochemically equivalent to the fats of mammals and no doubt they provide a rich source of energy for the developing seedling. Needless to say, the lighter the seed the greater its chance of being widely dispersed, and it is significant that, at this exceptional stage of their development when mobility (albeit in the passive sense of seed dispersal) has an important influence on their chance of survival, many plants rely heavily on the fatty acid system of storage.

In conclusion, we can now see that although the energy economy of the biosphere is founded on carbohydrate metabolism, fatty acids do make an important contribution and their metabolism is of great interest in the context of bioenergetics. In the following account we shall focus our attention on this aspect of their metabolism, beginning with the catabolic pathway.

The catabolic pathway

Scheme 10.3 shows in outline how stearic acid is degraded. Starting with the coenzyme A derivative of the fatty acid the chain is broken down, two carbon atoms at a time, by the repeated operation of a standard sequence of reactions to be given in detail later. Obviously, the degradation of an unsaturated acid has to follow a slightly more complicated course, because this standard sequence will have to vary at the stage when a double bond is reached, but in this account we shall ignore these minor variations and deal with the metabolism of saturated fatty acids only.

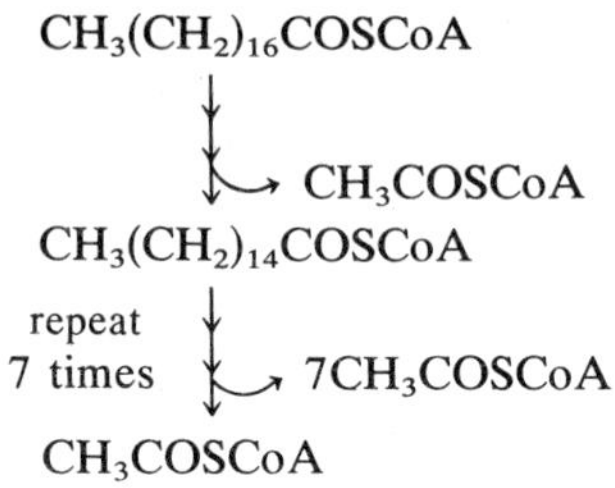

$$CH_3(CH_2)_{16}COSCoA$$

$$\downarrow \quad CH_3COSCoA$$

$$CH_3(CH_2)_{14}COSCoA$$

repeat
7 times $7CH_3COSCoA$

$$CH_3COSCoA$$

SCHEME 10.3

Each C_2 unit is released as acetyl CoA, including the final surviving residue, so that, in all, nine units of this compound are generated from one molecule of stearic acid. The process takes place in the mitochondrion and so the product is already in the correct compartment for further degradation via the citric acid cycle.

Prior to entering the degradation sequence the fatty acid is converted to its coenzyme A derivative and this is achieved by coupling the process to the hydrolysis of ATP. The coupled reaction takes the unusual form shown in Scheme 10.4 where the ATP is cleaved to AMP and pyrophosphate rather than ADP and phosphate. The advantage of this unusual mode of cleavage is that it leads to a greater driving force for thioester formation. This results not from the initial cleavage (the equilibrium constant for the isolated coupled reaction shown in Scheme 10.4 is, like those discussed earlier, close to unity), but from the subsequent thermodynamically favourable cleavage of the pyrophosphate to two molecules of phosphate (which takes place on a different enzyme). Overall two phosphoric anhydride bonds undergo cleavage in the formation of the thioester and the reaction goes virtually to completion.

The thioester is now ready for removal of the first C_2 unit by the sequence of reactions shown in Scheme 10.5. For convenience the scheme shows the penultimate cycle of operations in which hexanoate is degraded to butyrate.

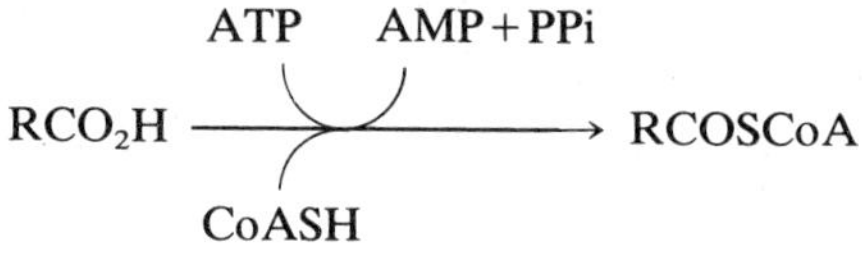

$$ATP \quad AMP + PPi$$

$$RCO_2H \longrightarrow RCOSCoA$$

$$CoASH$$

SCHEME 10.4

SCHEME 10.5. The pathway of fatty acid degradation.

$CH_3CH_2CH_2CH_2CH_2COSCoA$

(1)

$\begin{array}{c} \diagup FAD \\ \diagdown FADH_2 \end{array}$

(1) The flavoprotein which carries out this dehydrogenation is located in the mitochondrion and the process is closely related to the dehydrogenation of succinic acid to fumaric acid (step 7 of the citric acid cycle).

$CH_3CH_2CH_2CH\!\!=\!\!CHCOSCoA$

$\diagup H_2O$

(2) The newly introduced double bond is conjugated with a carbonyl group and so it is activated at the β-carbon towards nucleophilic attack by hydroxide ion or water. Consequently the step is related in mechanism to the hydration of fumaric acid (step 8 of the citric acid cycle).

$CH_3CH_2CH_2CHCH_2COSCoA$
$\qquad\qquad\quad |$
$\qquad\qquad\quad OH$

(3)

$\begin{array}{c} \diagup NAD^{\oplus} \\ \diagdown NADH \end{array}$

(3) This is a standard redox reaction in which the oxidation of an alcohol to a ketone is brought about by NAD^+.

$CH_3CH_2CH_2CCH_2COSCoA$
$\qquad\qquad\; \|$
$\qquad\qquad\; O$

(4)

$\diagup CoASH$

(4) The product of the previous step is a β-keto ester and in this key step it undergoes a characteristic cleavage between the α- and β-carbons. The fatty acid residue, now two carbons shorter, is released as its coenzyme A derivative and so it is ready for the next cycle.

$CH_3CH_2CH_2COSCoA + CH_3COSCoA$

repeat
steps
(1)–(4)

After repetition of steps (1)–(4) an acetate derivative is all that remains of the fatty acid chain and the degradation is complete.

$CH_3COSCoA + CH_3COSCoA$

Reaction mechanisms

The first three reactions of the sequence bring about the oxidation of a methylene group to a ketonic carbonyl group. The process is known as β-oxidation, in recognition of the fact that the methylene group involved is placed β to the ester goup, which provides the requisite activation at the appropriate stage. A mechanistic rationale for this type of transformation was presented in Chapter 8 during the discussion of the essentially equivalent conversion of succinic acid to oxaloacetate (steps 7–9 of the citric acid cycle) and so further comment is not required at this stage.

Turning to step (4), we meet a reaction which we have not considered in detail yet. It is of special interest as the key step of the sequence in which the fatty acid chain is broken. A possible mechanism based on analogy with the standard mode of β-keto ester cleavage is presented in Scheme 10.6.

Two separate units of coenzyme A take part in the mechanism and it is interesting to note that they serve in completely different roles. One unit participates directly by acting as a nucleophile in the first step and in doing so it triggers the cleavage step of the process. However, any other commonly used nucleophile could serve equally well in this capacity and so we have to look to the product of the last step to discover the advantage of using the thiol group of coenzyme A. Here we see that the shortened fatty acid residue is released as its coenzyme A derivative and thus it is already in the correct chemical form to enter the next cycle of operations.

The second unit of coenzyme A assists indirectly in the cleavage step. Here the carbonyl group of the thioester serves as a temporary sink for the electrons released from the breaking carbon-carbon bond and it will be more effective in performing this role when it is in the form of a thioester rather than that of an oxygen ester or the free acid.

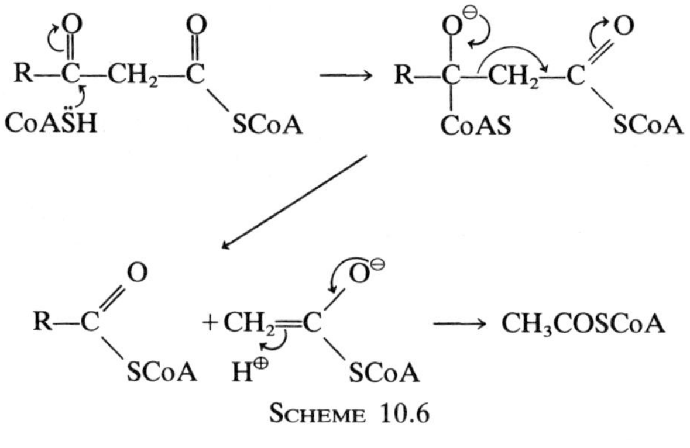

SCHEME 10.6

Bioenergetics

Bearing in mind that the reactions take place in the mitochondrion, it is reasonable to suppose that as a consequence of each cycle in which a C_2 unit is removed five units of ATP will be generated in the electron transport system. Three of these units would result in the usual way from the reoxidation of the NADH produced in step (3), and the remaining two units from the reoxidation of the flavoprotein that operates in the initial dehydrogenation of the fatty acid chain. However, it is not certain that the latter process is coupled to ATP production in the electron transport system; the suggestion that it will be so rests mainly on analogy with the closely related dehydrogenation of succinic acid during the course of the citric acid cycle.

Nevertheless we shall assume for the purpose of this discussion that five units of ATP are generated per cycle. This means that 40 units in all will be formed in the conversion of a molecule of stearyl CoA to nine of acetyl CoA. Each molecule of the latter will give rise to 12 units of ATP on passage through the citric acid cycle, making a further total of 108 units. On the other side of the balance sheet we have the loss of the equivalent of two units in the initial conversion of the free fatty acid to its thioester, so that the net yield of ATP arising from the complete combustion of a molecule of stearic acid (molecular weight 284) is 146 units. In comparison, glucose (molecular weight 180) yields only 38 units on total combustion.

Thus it can be calculated that, for a given weight of material, the recoverable energy content of a typical fatty acid is approximately two and a half times greater than that of glucose. In this figure we now have a quantitative measure of the considerable benefit gained by mammals from the practice of storing energy in the form of fats rather than carbohydrates and without doubt there has been strong evolutionary pressure on members of the animal kingdom to adopt this advantageous mode of storage. Nevertheless, it will seem ironic to some readers to see our ability to accumulate fat commended as a weight-saving measure, but perhaps those who need to watch their weight can draw some comfort from the thought that, were we to accumulate carbohydrate instead, the severity of their problem would be more than doubled!

To round off this section we need to consider the energetics of the reactions themselves in order to discover what are the factors that ensure that material traverses the pathway in the required direction. We have seen already that the initial step of thioester formation is given a powerful push by a special variant in which the equivalent of two units of ATP undergo hydrolysis. Passing on to the sequence of reactions shown in Scheme 10.5 we can identify steps (1) and (3) as reactions with a powerful driving force, not because of the inherent free-energy change, however, but as a result of the energy liberated when the respective coenzymes are reoxidized by molecular oxygen. Even allowing for the free energy harnessed in the form of ATP there will be a considerable surplus to be dissipated as heat in each case. In addition the equilibrium in step (4) strongly favours cleavage. Thus, three out of the four steps are favourable and so between them they will ensure that the remaining step proceeds in the required direction.

The anabolic pathway

The pathway of fatty acid biosynthesis is shown in outline in Scheme 10.7. Starting from acetate the chain is built up by the successive addition of C_2 units (chain building units) so that acetate is converted to butyrate, butyrate to hexanoate, and so on, until the required chain length is reached. In passing, it is interesting to note that only fatty acids having even numbers of carbons will be formed by this mode of synthesis.

The preparative strategy of the pathway is equivalent to a straight reversal of fatty acid degradation. However, in the details of its execution the synthesis differs from the degradation in several highly significant respects, and it is this fact that makes the comparison of the two so instructive.

Each extension of the chain is brought about by a fixed sequence of reactions and our main task is to analyse the chemical basis of the transformation. But first it is desirable to give a brief survey of the enzymology of the process to help set the chemistry in perspective.

In dealing with fatty acid degradation we could afford to ignore this aspect of the subject, apart from mentioning that the reactions take place in the mitochondrion, because the mode of operation of the enzymic

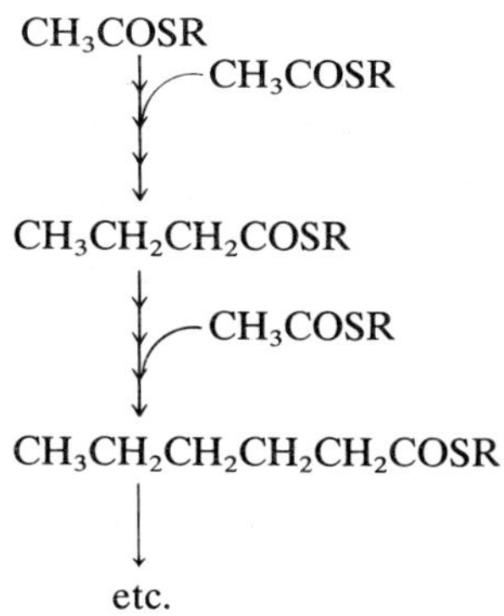

$$CH_3COSR$$

$$CH_3COSR$$

$$CH_3CH_2CH_2COSR$$

$$CH_3COSR$$

$$CH_3CH_2CH_2CH_2CH_2COSR$$

etc.

SCHEME 10.7

apparatus is relatively unexceptional. Thus each intermediate is present in the form of a coenzyme A derivative and having been formed on one enzyme it migrates through solution in the usual way until it reaches the enzyme that carries out the next step. In contrast the synthetic pathway shows a number of exceptional features in its enzymology and we shall examine two of them here.

First, all the individual enzymes of fatty acid synthesis are associated in the form of a multi-enzyme complex known as a fatty acid synthetase. From start to finish the growing fatty acid chain remains bound to the complex and there are no enzyme-free intermediates at any stage. Obviously this fact alone creates formidable difficulties for the investigator. In addition, the structure of the synthetase, and to a lesser extent its mode of action, varies according to the species of organism from which it is isolated. Therefore, in the following account we shall adopt as our model the synthetase isolated from the bacterium *E. Coli*. This is the one that is best understood at the present time and for the sake of simplicity we shall ignore the variations shown by synthetases isolated from other sources such as yeast or liver.

The second notable feature of the enzymatic apparatus of fatty acid biosynthesis concerns the nature of the thiol which acts as acyl carrier through the various steps of the pathway. This function is performed by coenzyme A in almost every area of metabolism including fatty acid catabolism, but in the biosynthesis of fatty acids the task is carried out by a special thiol designated ACP.SH. The initials ACP stand for acyl carrier protein, the full name of the compound, and as usual SH denotes the biologically active thiol group. [69] shows the partial structure of the compound in the vicinity of the active site, and it is intriguing to find there a unit of 4'-phosphopantotheine which is also present at the active site of coenzyme A. In the structure of the acyl carrier protein this residue is attached via its phosphate group to a serine unit of a protein chain. This chain contains 77 amino acid residues and it serves to bind the structure to the synthetase complex.

Protein chain

4'-Phosphopantotheine

[69]

When we consider the synthetic sequence in detail in Scheme 10.8 it will be clear that there must be two separate thiol binding sites, one to accommodate the chain starter unit (and in subsequent cycles the growing fatty acid), the other to bind the chain building unit. In the scheme both sites are shown as acyl carrier protein residues though this has not been established for certain. Initially two acetate units are transferred from the pool of acetyl CoA to the active thiol groups of the synthetase. These trivial steps are not shown in the scheme. The stage is now set for step (1) of the synthetic sequence. The product is a unit of butyrate. At the start of the next cycle this occupies the chain starter site and so is elaborated by the same sequence of steps to hexanoate. Eventually, when the requisite number of cycles have been completed, the free fatty acid is liberated from the enzyme by cleavage of the thioester link.

Preparative strategy

We are now in a position to appreciate how closely the anabolic pathway corresponds to a reversal of the steps of the catabolic pathway. This holds true particularly for the last three steps of the sequence, in which the keto group of a β-keto ester is reduced to a methylene, for this result is achieved by what is essentially a step by step reversal of the process of β-oxidation. Indeed the only significant difference in the chemical sense lies in the nature of the coenzymes which carry out the various hydrogen transfers, namely, $NADP^+/NADPH$ in the synthesis, and in the degradation, $NAD^+/NADH$ in cooperation with $FAD/FADH_2$.

The significance of this working arrangement was explained in the discussion of glucose biosynthesis and the only new point which needs to be mentioned here concerns the source of the hydrogen delivered by the NADPH. In a non-photosynthetic organism this cannot be specified other than to say that it will be derived from a range of metabolic redox reactions. The essential point will still apply however: the coenzyme couple will be maintained mainly in the reduced form and hence the redox reaction on the biosynthetic pathway will be driven in the required direction.

From every point of view the really intriguing stage of the synthetic sequence is the process by which the two thioesters are condensed to form a β-keto ester. In principle the synthetic pathway could have used the direct condensation process as shown in Scheme 10.9. As the direct reversal of the cleavage step of the catabolic sequence, this simple approach is certainly mechanistically feasible. However, it suffers from the serious disadvantage that the equilibrium point strongly favours cleavage and the effect of this adverse factor would accumulate on the addition of successive C_2 units. Nevertheless this mode of synthesis is not

Scheme 10.8. The steps of the synthetic sequence.

$CH_3COS.ACP$

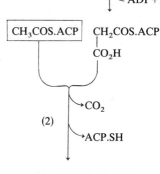

(1)   ⎧ ATP
       ⎩ ADP + Pi

(1) The chain building unit is converted to malonate by reaction with CO_2. Note that the process needs to be driven by ATP hydrolysis.

$\boxed{CH_3COS.ACP}$ $CH_2COS.ACP$
                         |
                         CO_2H

(2) This is the key step in which the chain starter unit (in the box) condenses with the chain building unit. The reaction is accompanied by decarboxylation of the carboxyl group.

(2)   → CO_2
       → ACP.SH

$CH_3COCH_2COS.ACP$

(3)   ⎧ NADPH
       ⎩ NADP+

(3) A standard reduction carried out by the nicotinamide coenzyme NADPH.

$CH_3CHCH_2COS.ACP$
    |
    OH

(4)   → H_2O

(4) The dehydration of a β-hydroxy acid is also standard.

$CH_3CH{=}COS.ACP$

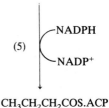

(5)   ⎧ NADPH
       ⎩ NADP+

(5) Another standard reduction carried out by NADPH.

$CH_3CH_2CH_2COS.ACP$

$$RCOSR' + CH_3COSR' \xrightarrow[R'SH]{} RCOCH_2COSR'$$

SCHEME 10.9

ruled out completely, for it does serve successfully in certain circumstances to bring about the extension of a fatty acid by one C_2 unit.

To overcome this hurdle, Nature has evolved steps (1) and (2) of the synthetic sequence which taken together constitute an ingenious roundabout route to achieve the desired transformation. These reactions make a fascinating study and accordingly we shall make a thorough examination of their bioenergetics and mechanism in the following sections.

Bioenergetics of steps (1) *and* (2)

For convenience the reactions are repeated in Scheme 10.10. In step (1) the chain building unit is converted from acetate to malonate. The latter then condenses in step (2) with the thioester of the fatty acid and in the process the newly introduced carboxyl group is lost. Our task then is to account for this apparently futile sequence of carboxylation followed by decarboxylation, for it holds the key to the condensation process. The significant feature of step (1), leaving aside the question of mechanism, is the fact that the process of carboxylation is coupled to the hydrolysis of ATP. This is necessary because of the unfavourable equilibrium of the unassisted reaction and it gives an indication of the free energy waiting to be liberated in the reverse reaction when the carboxyl group is lost. In step (2) this source of free energy is tapped by coupling the decarboxylation to the condensation and in this way the adverse energy barrier to the latter reaction is overcome. Therefore the carboxylated intermediate is in effect a high-energy derivative and the process as a whole represents an ingenious device for coupling the unfavourable condensation step to the hydrolysis of ATP. This strategy is not peculiar to fatty acid metabolism and we shall briefly examine

$$CH_3COS.ACP \xrightarrow[ATP \quad ADP + Pi]{CO_2 \quad (1)}$$

$$\overset{CO_2H}{|}\atop{CH_2—COS.ACP} \xrightarrow[CO_2 + ACP.SH]{RCOS.ACP \quad (2)} RCOCH_2COS.ACP$$

SCHEME 10.10

another example of its use later, but first we shall turn to the mechanism of steps (1) and (2).

Mechanism of steps (1) and (2): the coenzyme biotin

Before discussing the mechanism of carboxylation in step (1) it is necessary to introduce another coenzyme, biotin, which acts as catalyst. The structure of the coenzyme [70] shows the compound in its biologically active form bound to the enzyme via an amide link to a lysine residue of the protein chain.

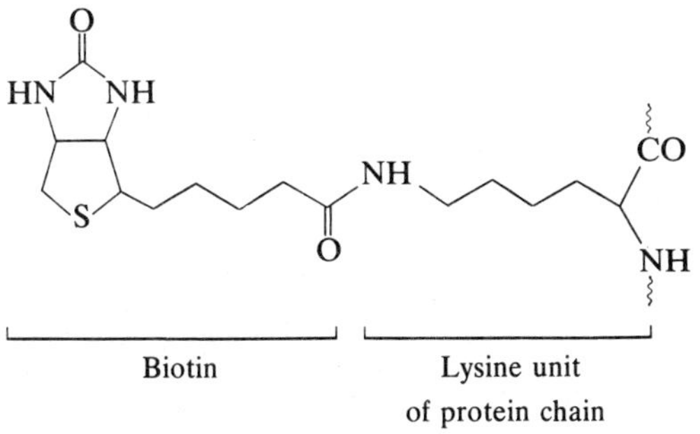

| Biotin | Lysine unit
                           | of protein chain |

STRUCTURE [70]

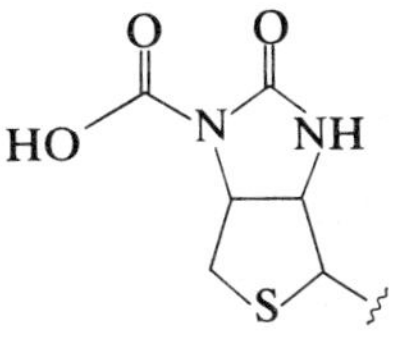

STRUCTURE [71] 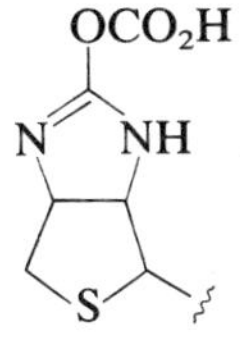   STRUCTURE [71a]

An important clue to the mode of action of biotin came from experiments in which enzyme–coenzyme complex was incubated with ATP and bicarbonate in the absence of substrate. A carboxylated derivative of the complex was formed which on controlled hydrolysis (after methylation with diazomethane) gave N-carboxybiotin [71] (as its methyl ester). It is possible therefore that the N-carboxy derivative of biotin is formed as an enzyme-bound intermediate in the normal metabolite reaction and that it transfers the carboxyl group to the carbanion derived from the substrate by a mechanism such as that shown in Scheme 10.11.

Scheme 10.12 shows a mechanism for the formation of the carboxylated intermediate in a way which accounts for the observation that one of the oxygen atoms of bicarbonate ion is transferred to the phosphate

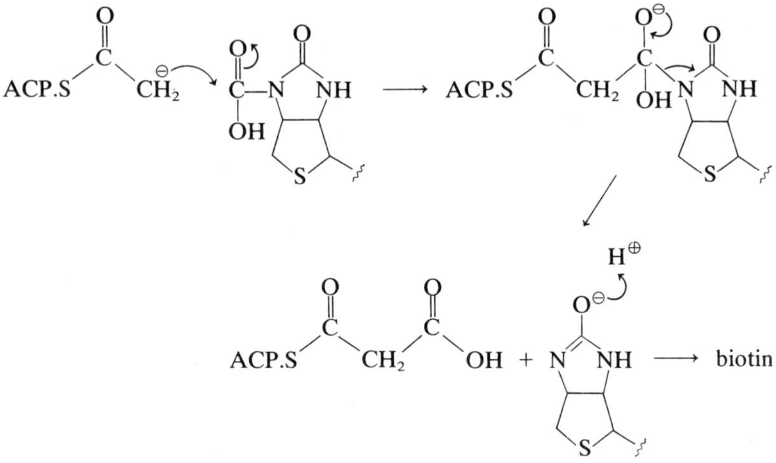

SCHEME 10.11

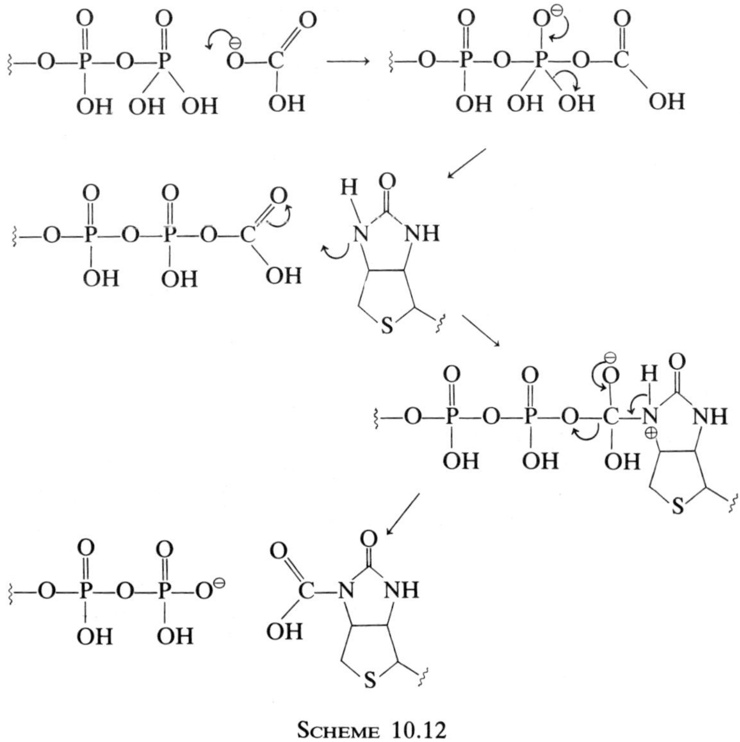

SCHEME 10.12

ion liberated from ATP. However, this simple mechanism involves the nitrogen atom of a urea in a nucleophilic role and it is therefore at variance with simple model experiments in which such atoms have proved to be embarassingly low in nucleophilic reactivity. A number of modified schemes have been advanced to overcome this objection. It has been suggested for example that the enzyme-bound intermediate might not be carboxylated on nitrogen as in [71] but on oxygen as in [71a]; the isolation of the N-carboxy derivative after hydrolysis could then be explained by an O to N migration of the acyl group in the course of the degradation. Hence the mechanism of action of biotin remains a challenging problem and the key to its solution may lie in further work on the structure of the enzyme-bound intermediate.

Turning to the carbon–carbon bond-forming step of fatty acid biosynthesis, we could consider a mechanism in which the reaction is initiated by deprotonation of the malonate to give a carbanion in the usual way. There is however an alternative, given in Scheme 10.13, in which the electrons required to generate the new carbon–carbon bond are made available by a concerted decarboxylation.

Whatever the mechanism of the condensation, the major advantage of carrying out the process by means of a carboxylation followed by decarboxylation is to be found in the sphere of bioenergetics. This ingenious device is not confined to fatty acid metabolism for we have already discussed briefly another example of its use in Chapter 3. The process in question was the conversion of pyruvate to phosphoenol pyruvate and it is worth discussing it further at this stage because it represents another important example of the use of biotin.

In the earlier account it was explained that the direct conversion, indicated by a dotted line in Scheme 10.14, is mechanistically feasible

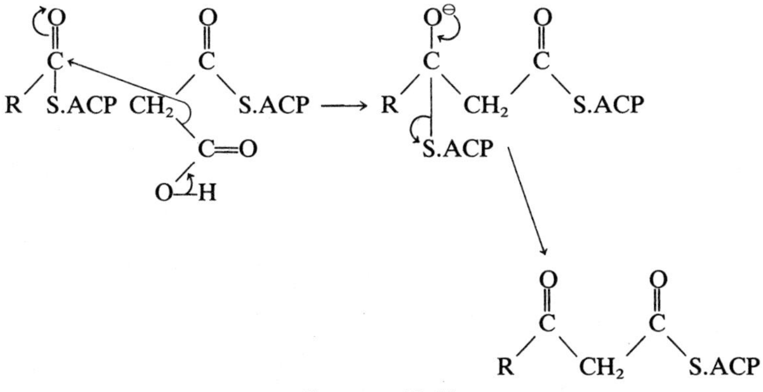

SCHEME 10.13

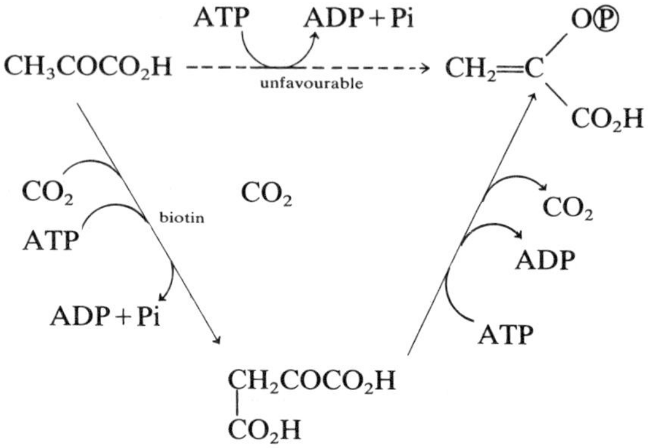

SCHEME 10.14

but that the adverse equilibrium renders the process useless as a method of preparation; indeed the reverse reaction is one of the favourable steps of the glycolytic pathway and as such it is an important source of ATP. To overcome this hurdle an indirect route is employed in which the pyruvate is carboxylated to give oxaloacetate. Once again this reaction is driven by ATP and biotin serves as a cofactor. The oxaloacetate then reacts with ATP, and, by undergoing a concerted decarboxylation in this step, it helps to drive the overall transformation in the desired direction.

A possible mechanism for the latter transformation is given in Scheme 10.15. Here again the decarboxylation provides the electrons to form the new bond, this time between an oxygen of oxaloacetate and the terminal phosphate of ATP.

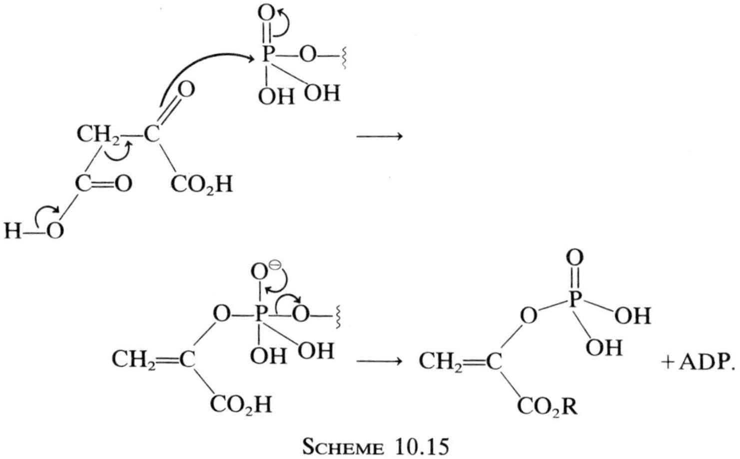

SCHEME 10.15

Factors which distinguish anabolism from catabolism

In fatty acid metabolism the anabolic pathway is very close to being a straightforward reversal of the catabolic pathway and consequently many of the intermediates are potentially common to both. The attendant risk that the two pathways might become crossed via a common intermediate must be avoided for obvious reasons.

The two pathways are kept separate in their operation by a number of factors. Firstly, there are those which help to differentiate the two processes in the chemical sense and so ensure that the enzymes of one pathway are not able to accept the intermediates of the other. In this connection one can cite (*a*) the use of two different thiols to act as carrier of the acyl group: coenzyme A for catabolism, the acyl carrier protein for anabolism; and (*b*) in the case of the β-hydroxy acid intermediates, an additional distinguishing feature not mentioned in the account: each of the β-hydroxy acid intermediates on the catabolic pathway has the *S*-configuration at the carbinol carbon whereas the corresponding intermediates of the anabolic pathway have the *R*-configuration at that centre. The chemical differentiation between the two processes is reinforced by factors which keep them physically separate. Most important in this connection is the fact that the two sets of enzymatic apparatus are located in different compartments of the cell (the catabolic enzymes are located inside the mitochondria and the anabolic enzymes outside) and consequently a membrane helps to prevent the two sets of intermediates from mixing.

While on the subject of physical controls it is worth pointing out that it is necessary to do more than just separate the two sets of enzymes in order to ensure that the fatty acid storage system works in an orderly way. The starting materials have to be supplied and products removed, which means that material in some form needs to be transported through the outer membrane of the mitochondria. In addition, it is necessary to have control mechanisms which can switch the two processes on and off independently according to the prevailing need. However, as explained in Chapter 1, these matters are essentially biological rather than chemical and so lie outside our brief.

Fatty acids and the storage of energy

When we consider fatty acid metabolism from the standpoint of energy storage the first point to note is the fact that energy is consumed in the course of the synthesis. This was not quantified in the account, but it can be calculated (on the basis that one unit of NADPH is equivalent to three of ATP) that, in effect seven units of the latter are used for each cycle of the synthetic sequence. However, it is not the consumption of ATP during the course of the synthesis that sets fatty acid metabolism apart from most other areas of metabolism and qualifies it to act as an energy storage system. Rather, it is the fact that free energy can be recovered in good yield to produce ATP during the course of the catabolic pathway. We saw earlier that as many as five units of ATP may be formed in each cycle, which means that up to 70 per cent of the energy put into store can be recovered for subsequent use. This represents a remarkably high level of recovery and it compares well with the chemical systems of energy storage devised by modern technology; needless to say, the Laws of Thermodynamics rule out the possibility of recovering 100 per cent of the stored energy in a system which is to be of practical value.

Even though the level of recovery is remarkably high, we must not overlook the fact that a significant proportion of the energy put into store in the form of a fatty acid is not recoverable. This loss is an important factor to be taken into account when comparing the relative merits of the two main systems of energy storage and it brings us back to the notable divergence between plant and animal metabolism in this respect. For we can now appreciate that when an animal converts carbohydrate to fat in the interests of saving weight, it does so at a price and, given that this price is one which the sedentary members of the plant kingdom have no incentive to pay, it is not surprising that they rely on the carbohydrate system rather than the fatty acid system for their normal requirements.

11. Metabolism of the C₁ pool: tetra-hydrofolic acid

IN SELECTING reactions for detailed discussion we have confined our attention so far to the central pathways of metabolism. The decision to restrict the choice of topic in this way stemmed from the desire to give a coherent treatment of bioenergetics. However, bioenergetics apart, the central pathways do not have a monopoly of the chemically interesting metabolic reactions as will now become clear when we turn out attention to other areas of metabolism. Needless to say, one consequence of this change of tack will be a shift in emphasis from bioenergetics to reaction mechanism.

In this chapter we shall cover an important area of metabolism in which C_1 building blocks are generated for use in a host of biosynthetic pathways. At the outset it should be explained that carbon dioxide, arguably the most important C_1 building block of all, will not be covered further here. Instead we shall only be concerned with the metabolism of C_1 units at three lower levels of oxidation, equivalent to formic acid, formaldehyde, and methanol. These form a discrete pool of intermediates, known as the C_1 pool, the members of which can be readily interconverted, and from which C_1 building blocks can be withdrawn when required for biosynthesis. The topic divides conveniently into two separate sections, the first dealing with the processes of interconversion of intermediates within the pool, and the second with the mechanics of C_1 transfer from the pool and accordingly this line of attack will be pursued in the following treatment.

The components of the C₁ pool

Structure and function of tetrahydrofolic acid (FH_4)

A new coenzyme, tetrahydrofolic acid (commonly represented by the symbol FH_4), plays a crucial role in the reactions under discussion and so it is best to start with an account of its structure and mode of action.

It can be seen from the full structure of the coenzyme [72], that it contains three structural elements. It should be mentioned that there are equivalent coenzymes which have essentially the same structure except that the glutamate unit (which is part of the non-operative residue) is replaced by a short peptide chain. These structural variants function in the same way as tetrahydrofolic acid itself (but with different enzymes).

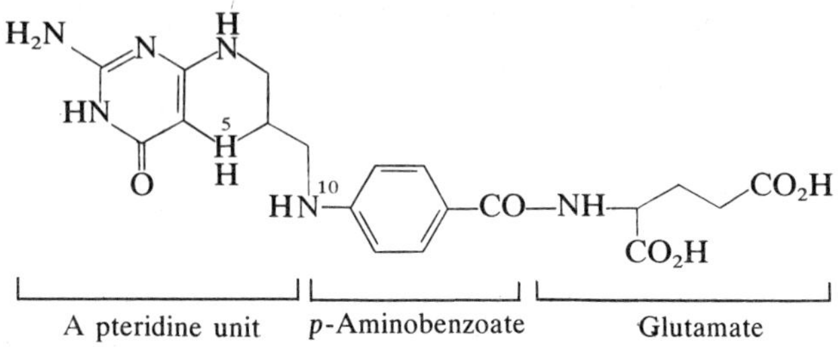

| A pteridine unit | *p*-Aminobenzoate | Glutamate |

[72]

Therefore, in the following account we shall treat all the coenzymes as one and not be concerned if, in a particular transformation, the active coenzyme is one of the variants rather than the parent coenzyme.

Tetrahydrofolic acid binds the C_1 unit by means of a covalent linkage to N^5 or N^{10} (and sometimes to both). Therefore the partial structure [73] will suffice for future representations of the coenzyme.

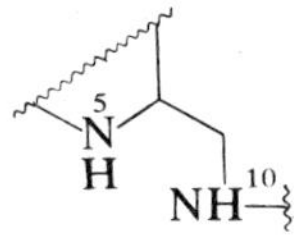

[73]

Tetrahydrofolic acid derivatives

The formate derivative. A C_1 unit at the formic acid level of oxidation can be bound to the enzyme in the form of an amide based on either N^5 as in [74] or N^{10} as in [75]. There is in addition a third derivative, [76], in which the C_1 unit is bound to both nitrogens simultaneously.

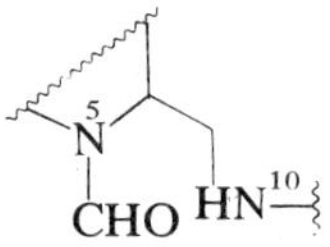

| N^5-formyl FH$_4$ | N^{10}-formyl FH$_4$ | N^5,N^{10}-methenyl FH$_4$ |
| [74] | [75] | [76] |

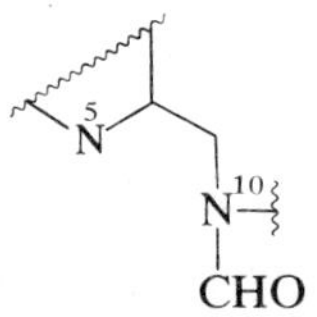

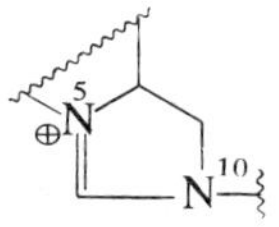

The main route by which formic acid enters the pool is illustrated in Scheme 11.1. Note that the condensation of free formic acid to form an amide derivative is coupled to the hydrolysis of ATP, and hence it provides another example of a thermodynamically unfavourable reaction which is driven in this way.

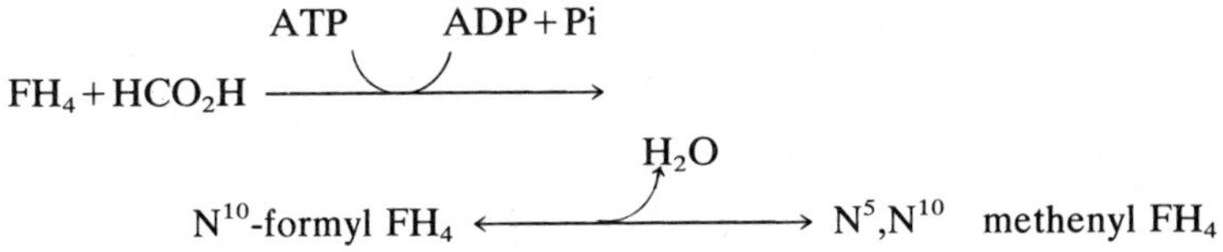

$$FH_4 + HCO_2H \xrightarrow{\quad \overset{ATP \quad ADP + Pi}{\underset{}{\bigvee}} \quad}$$

$$N^{10}\text{-formyl } FH_4 \xleftarrow{\quad \overset{H_2O}{\underset{}{\bigvee}} \quad} N^5,N^{10} \quad \text{methenyl } FH_4$$

SCHEME 11.1

The formaldehyde derivative. Scheme 11.2 shows the structure of the formaldehyde adduct [77], and as indicated it can be interconverted with free formaldehyde. A mechanism for the liberation of formaldehyde is given in Scheme 11.3.

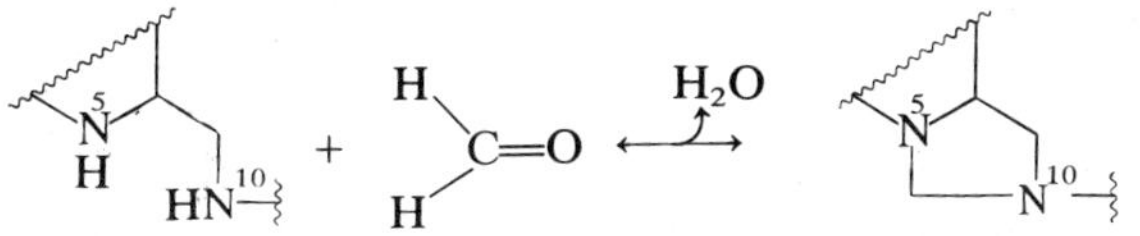

[77]

N^5,N^{10}-methylene FH_4

SCHEME 11.2

The methyl derivative. Although two methyl derivatives are possible in principle, only one [79] (based on N^5) is of importance in metabolism.

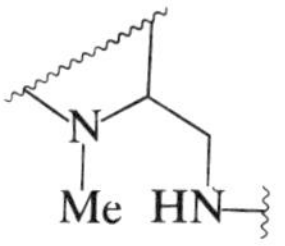

[79]

N^5-methyl FH_4

Redox reactions of the C₁ pool

We turn now to the interconversion of the various members of the C₁ pool. The requisite change in the oxidation level of the C₁ unit attached to tetrahydrofolic acid can be brought about by transfer of hydrogen to or from a nicotinamide coenzyme. The various redox transformations are

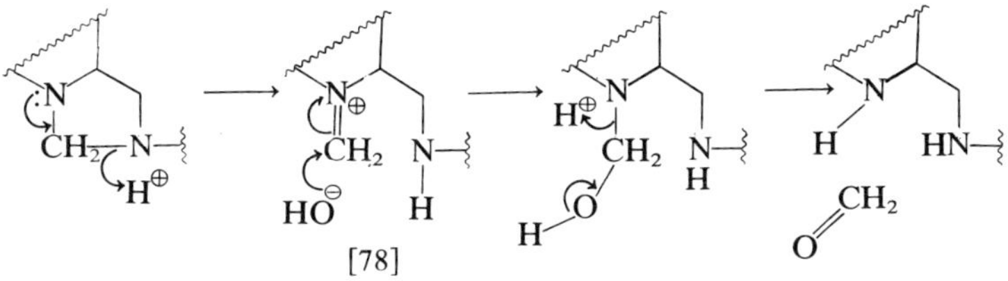

[78]

SCHEME 11.3

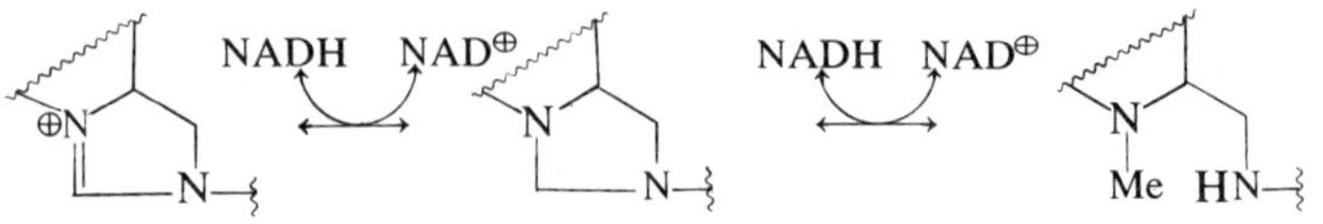

SCHEME 11.4

given in Scheme 11.4 and these reactions, together with those given earlier, provide a comprehensive network of pathways for the interconversion of C_1 units at the different levels of oxidation. Thus, for example, formic acid or formaldehyde can be used as a precursor of the methyl derivative of tetrahydrofolic acid and vice versa.

The mechanisms presented in Schemes 11.5 and 11.6 show the two reduction steps of Scheme 11.4 taking place by hydride attack on the carbon of the C_1 unit. Bearing in mind the discussion of the mechanism of action of NADH in Chapter 6 it will be clear that other mechanisms are open to consideration. However, it is noticeable that the reduction of the formate pool takes place on the cyclic derivative in which the C_1 unit will be at its most susceptible to nucleophilic attack by hydride transfer. With the same thought in mind it is suggested in Scheme 11.6 that the reduction of the formaldehyde derivative will take place on a ring-opened intermediate [78] (cf. Scheme 11.3). However, the latter process is complicated by the fact that it takes place with the assistance of a flavoprotein and so a radical mechanism must be considered a serious possibility.

Transfer of C_1 units from the C_1 pool

Formyl group transfer

Several reactions in which a unit of formate is transferred from the C_1 pool can be found on the pathways of biosynthesis. Generally speaking a

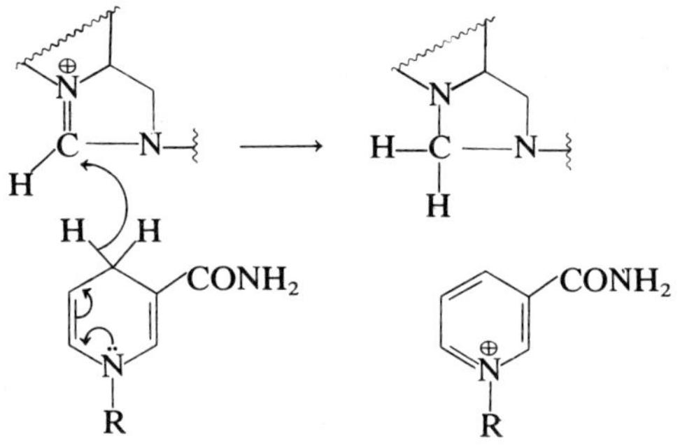

SCHEME 11.5

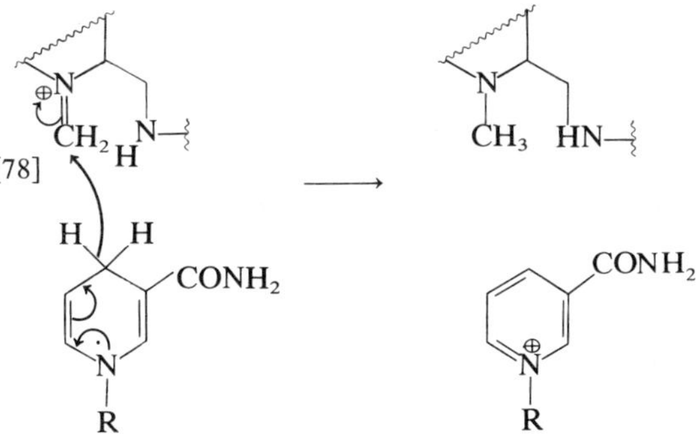

SCHEME 11.6

formyl group is exchanged from the nitrogen of the coenzyme to an equivalent group in the metabolic intermediate, presumably by one of the standard modes of acyl transfer. For example, this type of reaction takes place in the biosynthesis of the purines.

Transfer of a formaldehyde equivalent

There is only one reaction worthy of note in which the C_1 unit undergoes transfer at the formaldehyde level of oxidation and it takes place in the conversion of one amino acid, glycine [80], to another, serine [81]. The process is illustrated in Scheme 11.7. As indicated it is reversible, and so, given an adequate supply of serine, it can be used to provide material for the C_1 pool, or, alternatively, in the event of a deficiency of this amino acid, the C_1 pool can be used as a source of building blocks for its biosynthesis.

The mechanism of the transformation makes a fascinating study, but it does present a special difficulty because it involves a second coenzyme, pyridoxal phosphate (which we have not met yet) in a vital catalytic role. This coenzyme is of major importance and an account of its mode of action will be given in the next chapter. Fortunately, however, it is possible to cover the general principles of the mechanism of serine formation including the role of the tetrahydrofolate cofactor without knowing in detail how the second coenzyme achieves its catalytic effect.

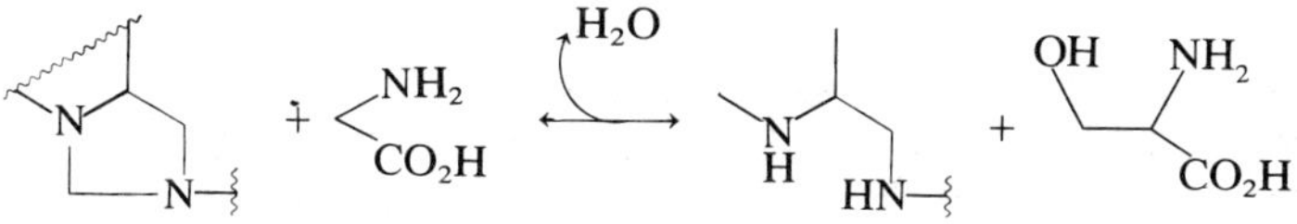

SCHEME 11.7

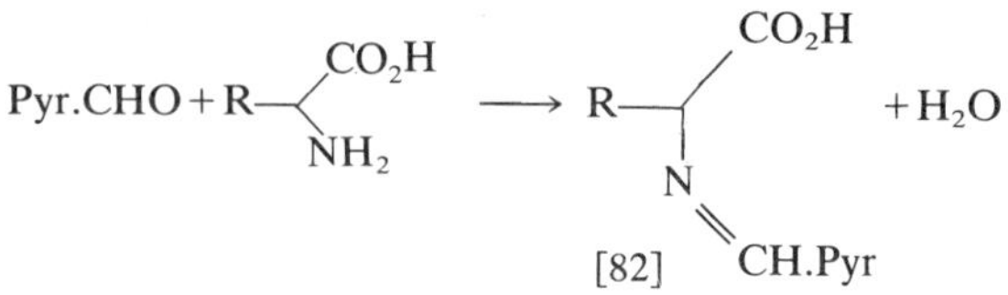

$$\text{Pyr.CHO} + \text{R} \underset{\text{NH}_2}{\overset{\text{CO}_2\text{H}}{<}} \longrightarrow \text{R} \underset{\underset{\text{CH.Pyr}}{\parallel}}{\overset{\text{CO}_2\text{H}}{\diagup}} + \text{H}_2\text{O}$$

[82]

SCHEME 11.8

In the following account, therefore, the mode of action of pyridoxal phosphate will be explained in outline only, so as to avoid anticipating too much of the subject matter of Chapter 12.

Pyridoxal phosphate contains a biocatalytically active aldehyde group which is conjugated with an aromatic ring. The constitution of the latter need not be specified at this stage and hence the structure of the coenzyme will be represented for the moment by Pyr.CHO. The coenzyme functions almost exclusively in the metabolism of the amino acids and its role is to assist the formation of a carbanion on the α-carbon of such compounds. It achieves this by condensation of its aldehyde group with the amine group of the substrate to generate an imine derivative [82], as in Scheme 11.8. The α-carbon is now strategically placed adjacent to an extended π-system, and, as a result, a carbanion formed at that site is considerably stabilized by delocalization with the aromatic ring of the coenzyme.

In the mechanism for serine formation, such carbanions are formed at no fewer than three steps. This is evident in Scheme 11.9 which starts with the carbanion [83], formed by deprotonation of the pyridoxal phosphate derivative of glycine. In step (1) this undergoes nucleophilic attack on the methylene derivative of tetrahydrofolic acid to form a carbon-carbon bond; for reasons explained in connection with Scheme 11.6 the tetrahydrofolate component is shown reacting in its ring-opened form. In step (2) the α-carbon is deprotonated a second time to give a stabilized carbanion [84], which then undergoes β-elimination in step (3) to remove the tetrahydrofolate cofactor. Nucleophilic attack of hydroxide on the alkene bond of [85] gives rise in step (4) to [86], the final carbanion in the scheme. This product is now recognizably a derivative of serine and all that remains to produce the free amino acid is a protonation step followed by hydrolytic removal of the pyridoxal phosphate.

Inevitably, the above account has important gaps with respect to the mode of action of pyridoxal phosphate but these will be filled in during the course of the next chapter. For the moment we shall concentrate on the role of the tetrahydrofolate. In this connection we need consider only the first three steps of the scheme, and their underlying rationale will be explained by analogy with the Mannich reaction.

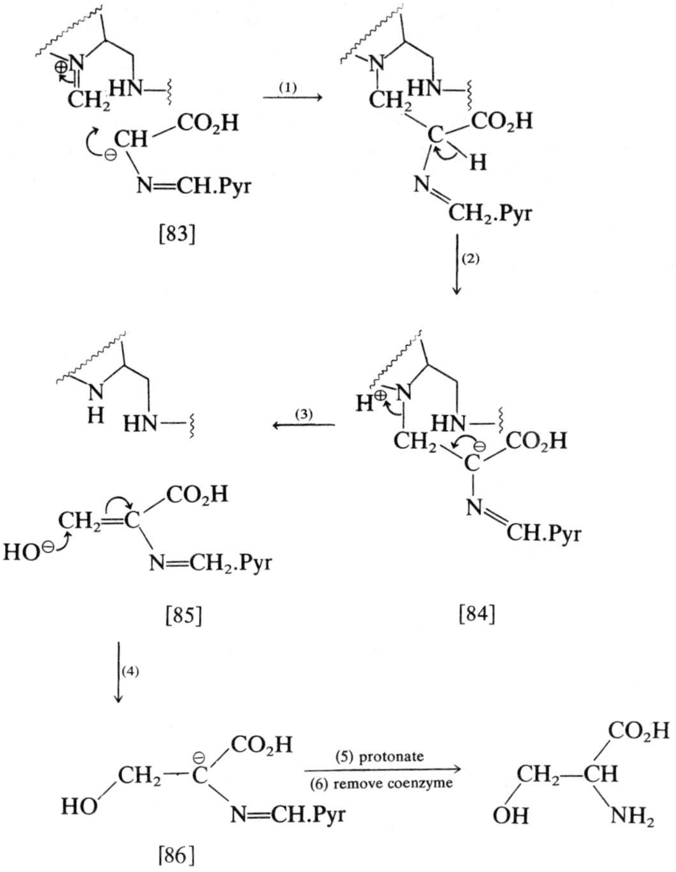

$$CH_2 \quad HN—\{$$
$$\overset{\ominus}{C} \quad CH \overset{CO_2H}{\diagdown} $$
$$N=CH.Pyr$$

[83]

$$\xrightarrow{(1)}$$

$$CH_2 \quad HN—\{$$
$$C \overset{CO_2H}{\underset{H}{\diagdown}}$$
$$N \overset{}{=} CH_2.Pyr$$

$$\downarrow (2)$$

$$\xleftarrow{(3)} \quad H^{\oplus} N$$
$$CH_2 \overset{\ominus}{C} CO_2H$$
$$N \overset{}{=} CH.Pyr$$

[84]

$$H \quad HN—\{$$

$$CH_2 = C \overset{CO_2H}{\diagdown}$$
$$HO^{\ominus} \qquad N = CH_2.Pyr$$

[85]

$$\downarrow (4)$$

$$CH_2 — \overset{\ominus}{C} \overset{CO_2H}{\diagdown}$$
$$HO \qquad N = CH.Pyr$$

[86]

$$\xrightarrow[\text{(6) remove coenzyme}]{\text{(5) protonate}}$$

$$CH_2 — CH \overset{CO_2H}{\diagdown}$$
$$OH \qquad NH_2$$

SCHEME 11.9

The latter is an important reaction in organic synthesis and a typical example, the synthesis of methyl vinyl ketone, is shown in Scheme 11.10. The mechanism is given in Scheme (11.11), which begins with the catalyst, dimethylamine, condensing with the formaldehyde to give an imminium derivative (by a mechanism of a standard type and therefore not shown), This intermediate is subjected to nucleophilic attack by the carbanion derived from acetone (step 1). Then a second carbanion is formed (step 2) which triggers the elimination of the catalyst in step (3). In this process the catalytic role of the amine is based on two principles: firstly, it is used to generate an imminium derivative which has the advantage of being more susceptible to nucleophilic attack than the free

$$H_2CO + CH_3COCH_3 \xrightarrow{\text{Me}_2\text{NH}} H_2C{=}CHCOCH_3 + H_2O$$

Scheme 11.10

aldehyde; secondly, it can serve as a satisfactory leaving group in step (3). If we now compare this mechanistic scheme with that advanced for serine formation it is immediately clear that each step of the chemical reaction is equivalent in its mechanism to the correspondingly numbered step in the biological reaction. Hence it is arguable that the catalytic activity of the tetrahydrofolate coenzyme is, like that of methylamine, based on the two principles mentioned above. However, one needs to tread with caution here because, as we shall see in the next chapter, the type of transformation that is involved in serine formation can take place without the assistance ot tetrahydrofolate.

Methyl group transfer fron N-methyltetrahydrofolate

In contrast to the relatively restricted use of formate and formaldehyde, the methyl group is a very widely used biosynthetic building block and the C₁ pool based on tetrahydrofolic acid provides a major source of the material used in this way. In view of this, it is surprising that the methyl derivative of tetrahydrofolic acid is used in only one methyl transfer of any consequence and that is the methylation of one amino acid, homocysteine [87] to produce another, methionine [88].

As will be apparent from Scheme 11.12, the methyl group is simply transferred from nitrogen to sulphur. However, simple though it may appear on the surface, this process is most puzzling from the point of view of mechanism. It is tempting to postulate a straightforward S_N2 reaction in which sulphur attacks the methyl group. However, the nitrogen of the coenzyme would be a very poor leaving group in such a mechanism. Admittedly the reaction might be assisted on the enzyme by prior protonation of the leaving group. However, nitrogen shows poor

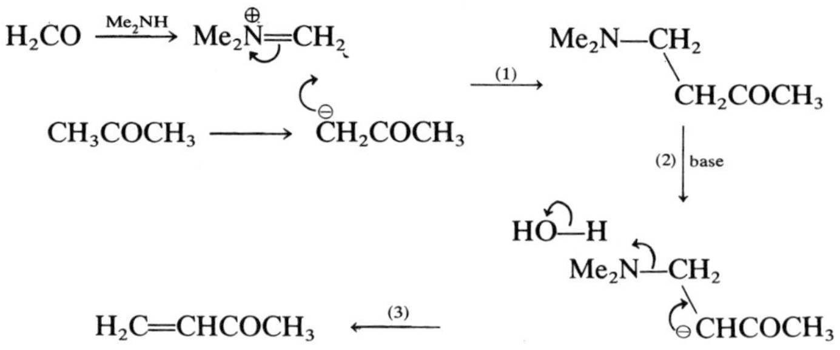

Scheme 11.11

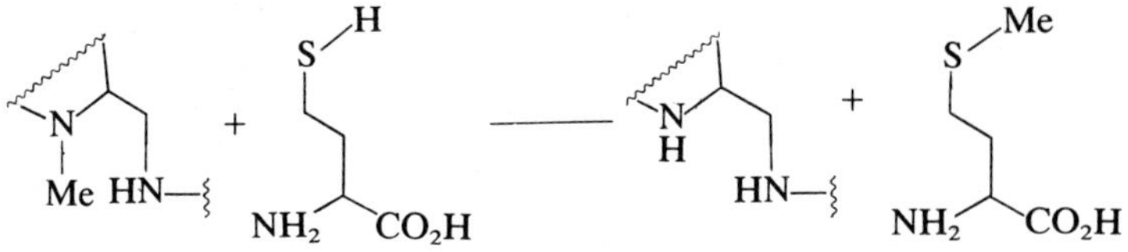

SCHEME 11.12

leaving ability even when in the form of a quaternary derivative so the proposed S_N2 reaction must still be viewed with caution.

Methionine as the ubiquitous methyl donor

The methione formed in this way now serves in turn as the general methyl donor in a host of biosynthetic reactions. The way in which it does so has been extensively studied and the general principles of its operation are well understood. The amino acid is converted first to a sulphonium derivative, S-adenosylmethionine [89] by reaction with ATP. As far as the latter coenzyme is concerned this is an exceptional transformation for in it ATP serves as an alkylating agent rather than as a phosphorylating agent. Presumably the reaction takes place by the mechanism presented in Scheme 11.13 where the sulphur of the methionine undergoes nucleophilic attack on one of the carbons of ATP (the methylene of the adenosyl residue; see [89]). The leaving group, trimetaphosphate, is a good one and the process is favourable. As a result the methionine is converted to a high-energy derivative in which the sulphur is now potentially a good leaving group and so the methyl is readily transferred to a suitable nucleophile, X^-, by S_N2 attack as in the final step of Scheme 11.13.

As is usual in this sort of process a cyclic pattern of operations can be envisaged and the full cycle is shown in Scheme 11.14. Here the

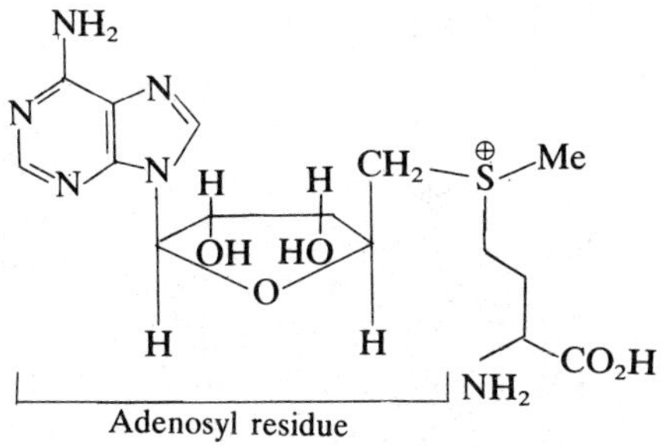

[89]

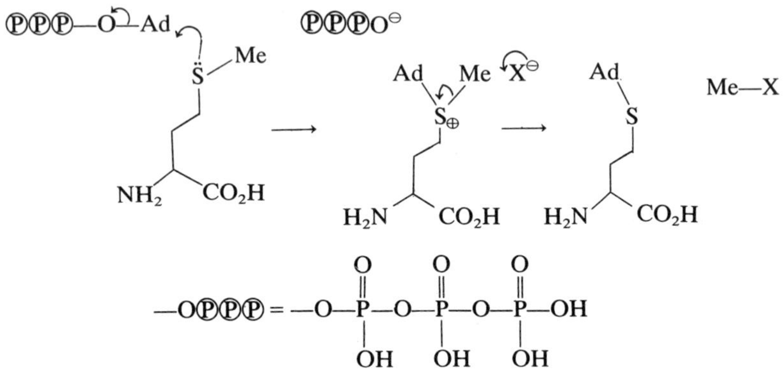

Scheme 11.13

by-product of the methylation step, S-adenosylhomocysteine [90], is hydrolysed to adenosine (AdOH) and homocysteine. The former is recycled to ATP; the latter returns to the C_1 pool to pick up a methyl group for the next cycle.

Thus the methionine functions in effect as a carrier to deliver methyl groups from the C_1 pool based on tetrahydrofolic acid to the host of acceptors represented by X^-. The list of acceptors includes compounds with nucleophilic carbon (e.g. enolate or alkene), nucleophilic oxygen (e.g. carboxylate, enolate, or phenolate), nucleophilic nitrogen, and nucleophilic sulphur.

Vitamin B_{12} and methyl transfers

It would be remiss to close this account without mentioning that another coenzyme, derived from vitamin B_{12}, has been implicated in

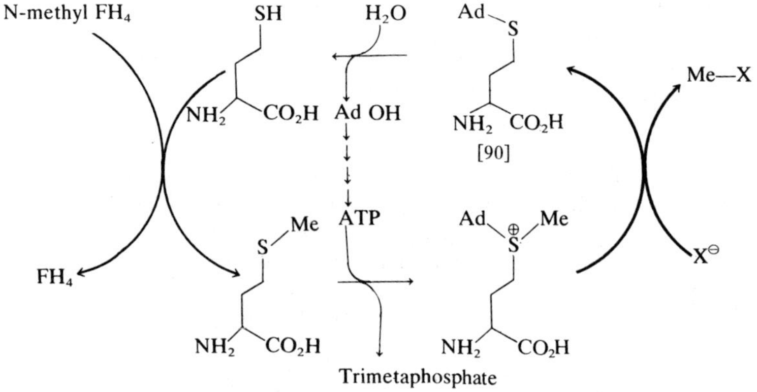

Scheme 11.14

methyl transfer metabolism. Very little is known about the process at present, but there is good evidence for the formation of an intermediate in which the methyl group is bound to the coenzyme via a covalent link to cobalt, and that it is then transferred from the metal to an acceptor. Clearly this is a remarkable process. Further investigation should reveal some fascinating and unexpected chemistry and the same holds for several other aspects of methyl group metabolism.

12. Amino acid metabolism and pyridoxal phosphate

THE DECISION to cover amino acid metabolism in this highly selective book can be justified on a number of grounds: firstly, because the catabolic pathways in this area provide an important source of energy in many organisms; secondly, because the amino acids themselves are essential as the building blocks from which enzymes are made; and thirdly, because this area of metabolism sees the operation of pyridoxal phosphate which is arguably the most fascinating of all the coenzymes on our brief.

Given that there are more than twenty essential amino acids it is clearly not possible in the space available to consider the metabolism of each one step by step. Instead we shall concentrate on the various types of transformation which hinge on the primary amino group, for these are the reactions which form the distinctive feature of amino acid metabolism. As we shall see they rely almost invariably on the catalytic effect of pyridoxal phosphate. Therefore in the following account we shall cover the mechanism of action of this coenzyme first and then examine a few selected amino acid pathways to see how they fit into the metabolic pathways map.

Reactions catalysed by pyridoxal phosphate

Representative examples of the various types of reaction catalysed by pyridoxal phosphate are shown in Scheme 12.1. One feature which stands out immediately is the extraordinary diversity of the reactions which range from carbon–carbon bond formation and cleavage (reactions 1 and 3), through examples of carbon-nitrogen bond formation and cleavage (e.g. reactions 7 and 8) and various redox transformations (reactions 5, 6, 7, and 8), to a reaction (number 4) in which one hetero-atom is displaced by another.

The varied nature of these reactions makes the study of their mechanism a formidable challenge. As we shall see all the reactions can be rationalized in terms of mechanism. Moreover though they vary in detail all the mechanistic schemes are based on the same mechanistic strategy. The unifying rationale which emerges can be considered a triumph for the mechanistic approach, and this subject therefore provides a fitting climax to our survey of coenzyme mechanisms.

SCHEME 12.1. Reactions catalysed by pyridoxal phosphate.

(1) Decarboxylation

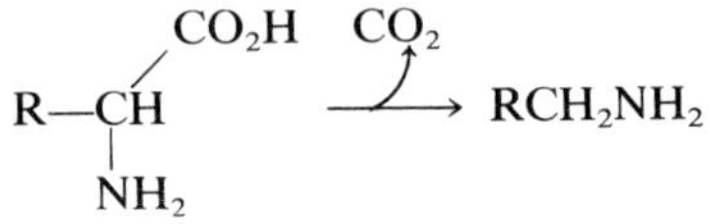

$$R-\underset{\underset{NH_2}{|}}{CH}\diagup^{CO_2H} \xrightarrow{\quad CO_2 \quad} RCH_2NH_2$$

(2) Racemization

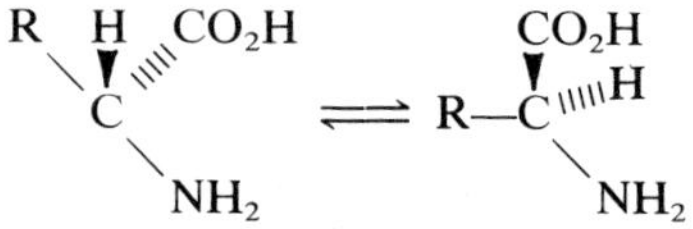

$$\underset{NH_2}{\overset{R\ H\ CO_2H}{C}} \rightleftharpoons R-\underset{NH_2}{\overset{CO_2H}{C}}\text{\tiny{IIIIH}}$$

(3) Carbon–carbon bond formation

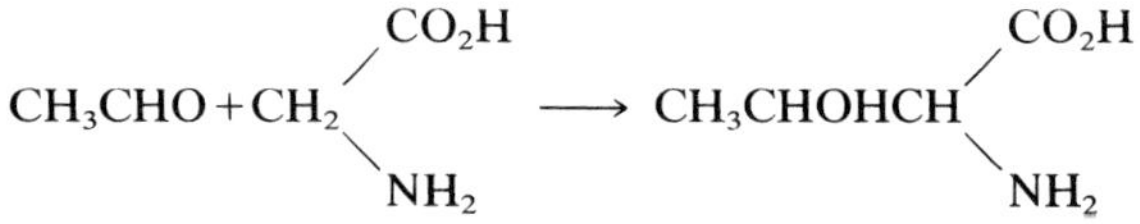

$$CH_3CHO + CH_2\diagup^{CO_2H}_{\diagdown NH_2} \longrightarrow CH_3CHOHCH\diagup^{CO_2H}_{\diagdown NH_2}$$

(4) Displacement at the β-carbon

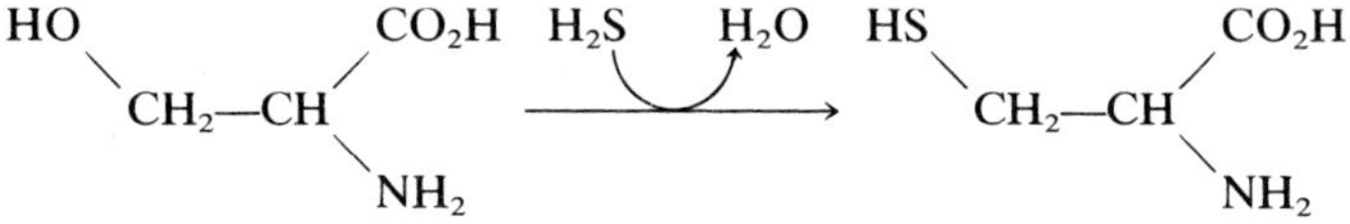

$$\underset{\diagdown CH_2-CH\diagdown NH_2}{HO}^{CO_2H} \xrightarrow[\quad H_2S \quad H_2O \quad]{} \underset{\diagdown CH_2-CH\diagdown NH_2}{HS}^{CO_2H}$$

(5) Internal redox reactions: between C_α and C_β

$$\underset{\overset{\beta}{CH_2}-\overset{\alpha}{CH}\diagdown NH_2}{HO}{}^{CO_2H} \xrightarrow[\quad H_2O \quad NH_3 \quad]{} CH_3COCO_2H$$

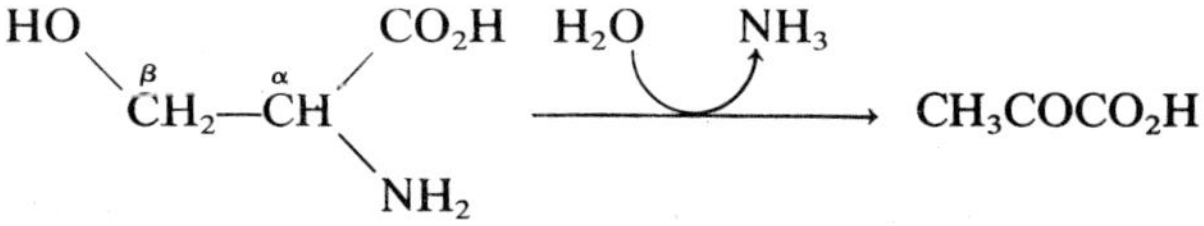

(6) Internal redox reactions: between C_α and C_γ

$$\underset{\overset{\gamma}{CH_2}CH_2\overset{\alpha}{CH}\diagdown NH_2}{HS}{}^{CO_2H} \xrightarrow[\quad H_2O \quad H_2S \quad NH_3 \quad]{} CH_3CH_2COCO_2H$$

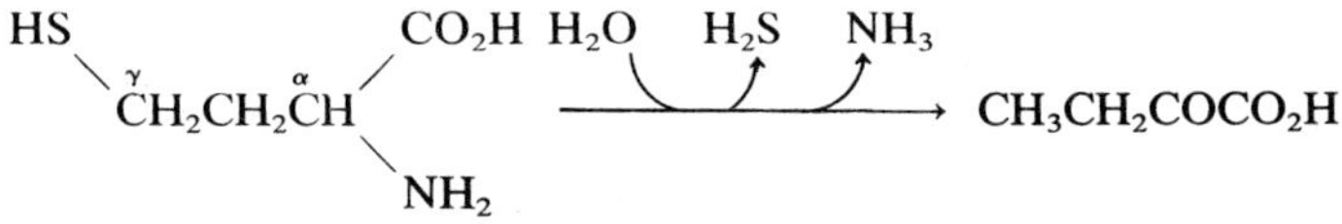

(7) Interconversion of an α-amino acid and α-ketoacid

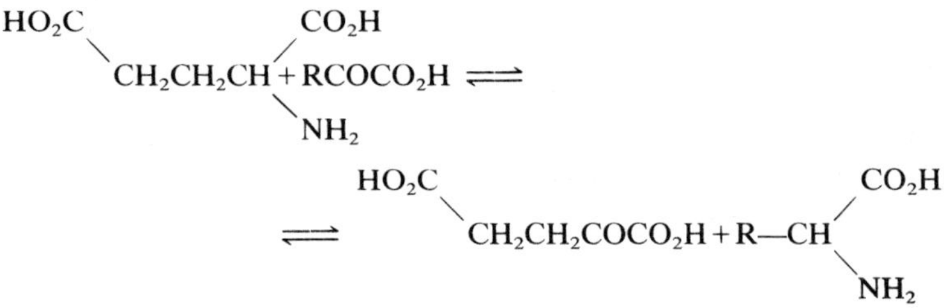

$$\underset{\diagdown CH_2CH_2CH\diagdown NH_2}{HO_2C}{}^{CO_2H} + RCOCO_2H \rightleftharpoons$$

$$\rightleftharpoons \underset{\diagdown CH_2CH_2COCO_2H}{HO_2C} + R-CH\diagup^{CO_2H}_{\diagdown NH_2}$$

Scheme 12.1 (Continued)

(8) Oxidation of a primary amine

$$RCH_2NH_2 \xrightarrow[\text{H}_2\text{O}]{\substack{O_2 \quad H_2O}} RCHO + NH_3$$

Structure of pyridoxal phosphate

The structure of the coenzyme is given in diagram [91]. Several compounds closely related in structure have been isolated from natural sources but with one exception these structural variants have proved to be devoid of biocatalytic activity. One interesting example is pyridoxal [92]. This is totally inactive even though it differs from the coenzyme solely in its lack of the phosphate group. However, it is not thought that the latter group is an active participant in the catalytic mechanism but rather that it plays an essential part in the process of enzyme recognition and binding.

The only structural variant which can serve as a cofactor is pyridoxamine [93]. Even this compound is not an alternative to pyridoxal phosphate but is formed from the parent coenzyme as an intermediate in certain types of enzyme-mediated reaction.

Mode of action of the coenzyme

We have already seen in outline in the last chapter how the coenzyme achieves its catalytic effect. First the aldehyde group of the coenzyme condenses with the primary amino group of the substrate; in the resulting imine the aromatic ring of the coenzyme serves as an electron sink and so assists the formation of a carbanion on the α-carbon of the amino acid residue. From the full structures of a typical imine [94] and the corresponding carbanion [95] we can now appreciate how well fitted the coenzyme is to perform its allotted task. Thus the aldehyde group is strategically sited at C-4 of the pyridine ring, shown in the protonated form in [94], and hence the carbanion centre in the intermediate [95] is ideally placed to achieve maximum delocalization by interacting through the π-system with the positively charged nitrogen as shown. Indeed, it can be argued, so favourable is this delocalization, that the alternative canonical form, the extended enamine [96], is the more appropriate representation of the structure of the intermediate and that it should be used in the mechanistic schemes to follow. For example Scheme 12.2 shows how the mechanism for protonation of the α-carbon would be represented on the enamine form. However, in order to portray the intermediate as an enamine it is necessary to write out the structure of

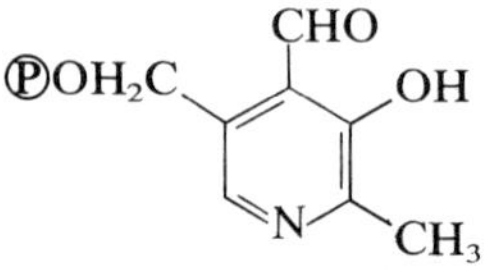

Pyridoxal phosphate
[91]

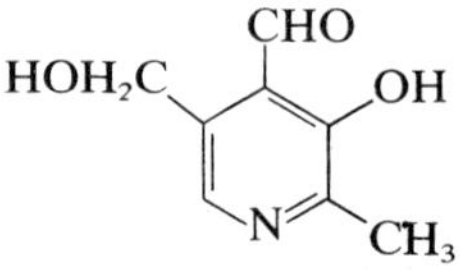

Pyridoxal
[92]

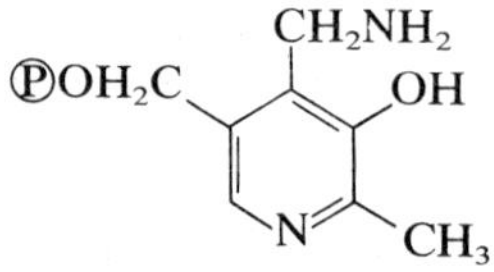

Pyridoxamine
[93]

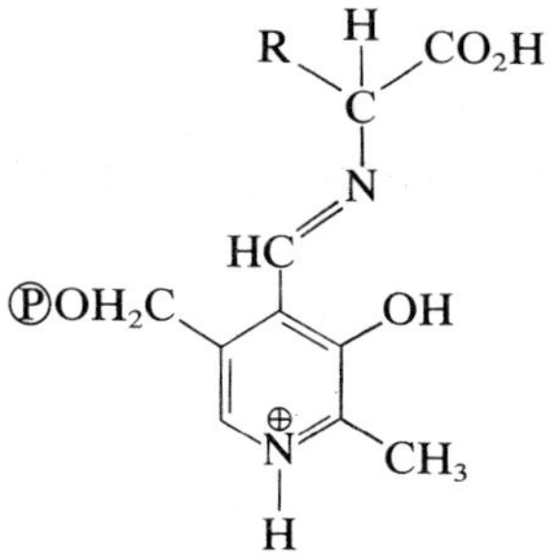

[94]

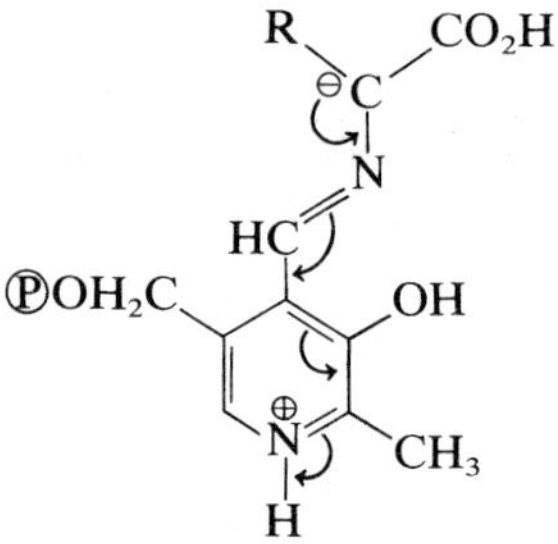

[95]

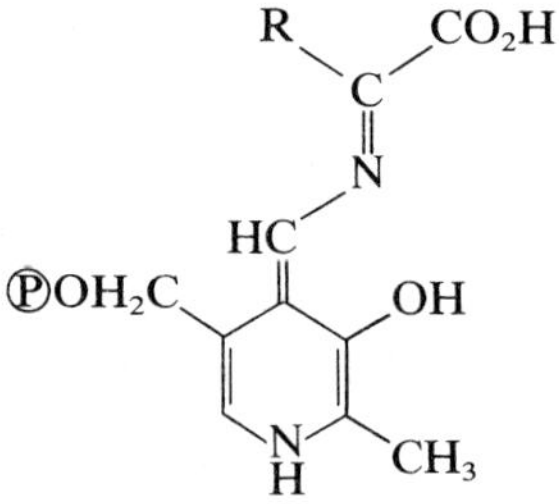

[96]

the coenzyme residue in full at every step of a mechanistic sequence. Therefore, in the following account we shall follow the practice established in the last chapter, where the coenzyme was represented by the abbreviation PyrCHO and the intermediates were portrayed as carbanions. In addition to saving space this practice has the merit that the diagrams are less complicated and attention is focussed on those electronic shifts which will be our main interest from now on, that is, those which take place in the substrate and thereby differentiate one type of transformation from another.

Before going on to consider the various mechanistic schemes in full it is convenient to consider two stages which are common to them all. These are the initial step which sees the formation of the key imine

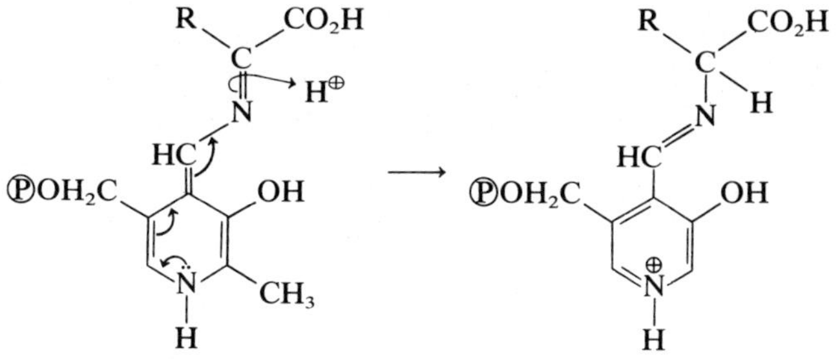

SCHEME 12.2

derivative of the substrate and coenzyme, and the final step in which an equivalent derivative of product and coenzyme is broken down. The former process does not take place, as might be expected, by direct condensation of the substrate amino group with the aldehyde group of pyridoxal phosphate. The reason for this is that the coenzyme does not exist as a free aldehyde when bound to the enzyme but exists instead as an imine [97] formed by condensation of the carbonyl group of the coenzyme with the primary amino group of a lysine unit of the protein chain (Scheme 12.3). Consequently, when the substrate, RNH_2, binds to the enzyme its imine derivative of the coenzyme must be formed by transimination as shown in Scheme 12.4. A similar transimination (but in the reverse sense) takes place at the end of each reaction scheme, with the result that the product is free to dissociate from the enzyme and the coenzyme is ready to react with the next molecule of substrate. The two transimination reactions will not be shown in the reaction schemes to follow.

It is interesting to speculate what advantage might be gained from the involvement of the amino group of lysine. Obviously the binding of the coenzyme will be assisted; we have already seen how lysine serves in a similar way to bind biotin to various enzymes. However, in the case of pyridoxal phosphate it is possible that the involvement of the lysine residue may also have a beneficial effect on the kinetics of the enzyme-mediated reaction, for it may result in a higher rate of formation of the

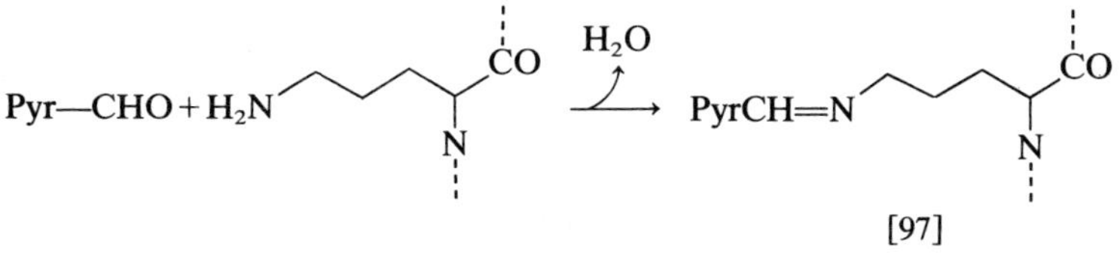

[97]

SCHEME 12.3

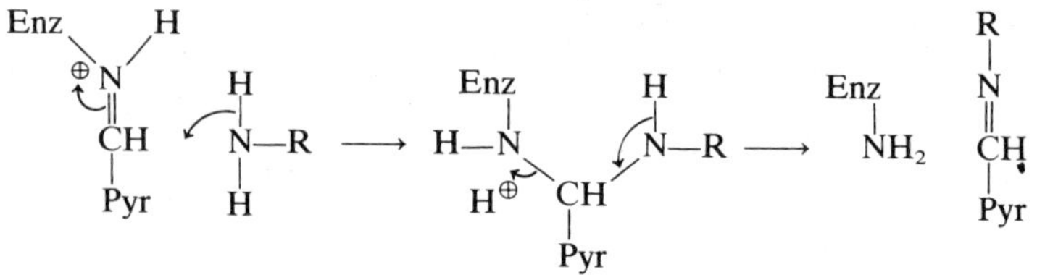

SCHEME 12.4

imine derivative of the substrate at the start of a transformation or, possibly, a more rapid breakdown of the corresponding derivative of the product in the final step.

Mechanism of decarboxylation and racemization

A plausible mechanism to account for the enzyme-mediated decarboxylation of an amino acid is given in Scheme 12.5. Scheme 12.6 shows how racemization might occur.

The two schemes are very closely related: each involves the formation of an intermediate carbanion which is then protonated. These mechanisms are based mainly on analogy with large numbers of related model reactions, many of which have been extensively investigated. For example, treatment of an amino acid with pyridoxal [92] in the presence of a trivalent metal cation at 100° results in competing racemization and decarboxylation of the starting material (other reactions can take place concurrently depending on the reaction conditions and the detailed structure of the compound under investigation). It has been shown that the two transformations under consideration take place by the mechanisms proposed for the equivalent enzyme-mediated reactions in Schemes 12.5 and 12.6. The role of the trivalent metal in the model reactions is particularly interesting. It is probable that a chelate is formed [98], which will have the advantage of holding the molecule in a favourable orientation for carbanion stabilization, that is with the p-orbitals of the imine π-bond parallel to those on the atoms of the aryl ring.

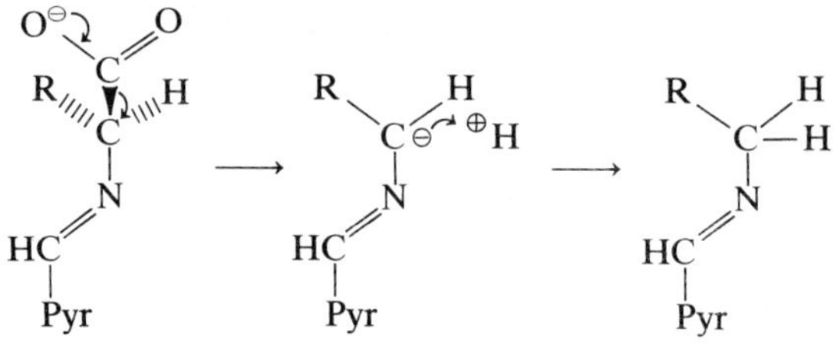

SCHEME 12.5

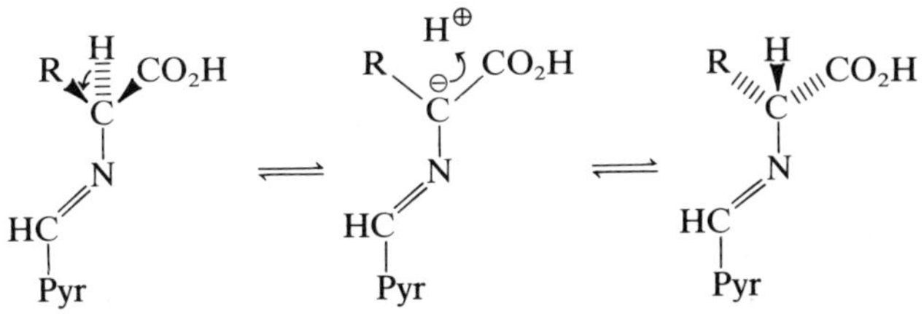

SCHEME 12.6

The fact that both racemization and decarboxylation take place in competition in this model reaction is in marked contrast to the absolute specificity of the various enzyme-mediated reactions. Presumably the nature of the reaction which takes place on a particular enzyme will be determined by the orientation of the substrate with respect to the various catalytic groups. Of particular importance in this respect is the conformation of the amino acid residue about the C_α–N bond in the imine intermediate. For maximum delocalization to take place in the transition state leading to the formation of the carbanion intermediate, the σ-bond to be cleaved must be coplanar with the p-orbital on the nitrogen of the imine. Presumably the shape of the active site of the enzyme will constrain the substrate in the required orientation: the two favourable orientations for proton removal were indicated in Scheme 12.6 and that for carboxyl loss in Scheme 12.5. In a model reaction on the other hand there will be relatively free rotation about the C_α–N bond (in contrast to the aforementioned restricted rotation about the σ-bond linking the imine residue to the aryl ring), and so either the hydrogen or the carboxyl group can achieve the favoured orientation for bond cleavage.

Mechanism of the carbon–carbon bond-forming reactions

In several of the biological reactions catalysed by pyridoxal phosphate the intermediate carbanion functions as a nucleophile towards carbon

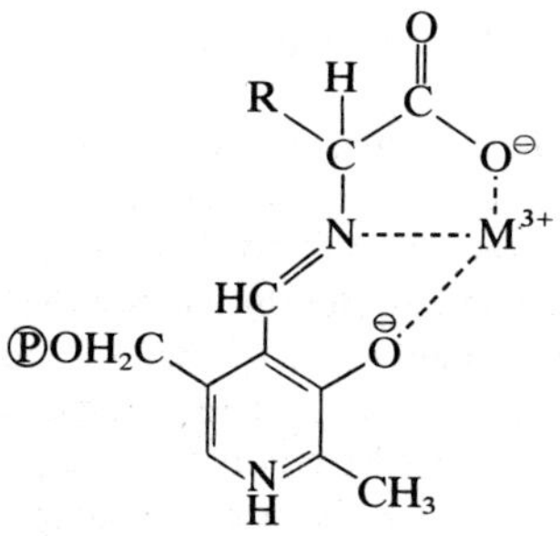

[98]

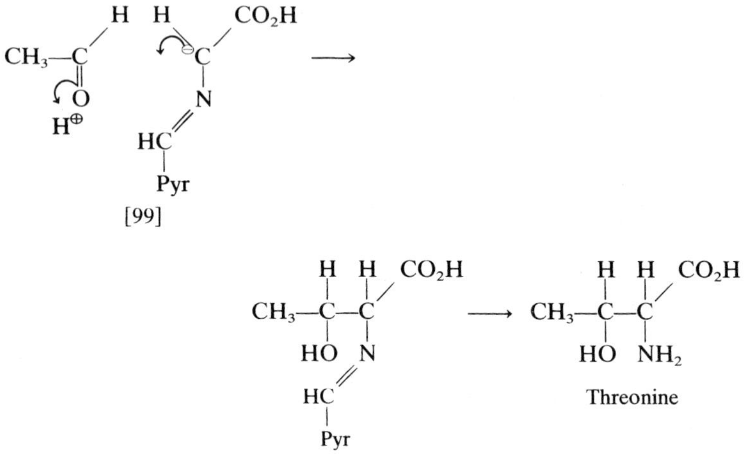

[99]

Threonine

SCHEME 12.7

instead of accepting a proton. Three examples are discussed below, two of which involve attack on carbon at the aldehyde level of oxidation, the third on a carboxylic acid derivative.

Formation of threonine. One of the biosynthetic routes to this essential amino acid involves condensation of glycine with acetaldehyde as in reaction (3) of Scheme 12.1. The proposed mechanism, presented in Scheme 12.7, involves the usual intermediate carbanion undergoing nucleophilic attack on the carbonyl group of acetaldehyde. The process is readily reversible and when considered in the reverse direction it can be regarded as being complementary to the processes of racemization and decarboxylation shown in Schemes 12.6 and 12.5, in the sense that the carbanion intermediate is generated here by cleavage of the third σ-bond at the α-carbon of an amino acid.

Serine formation. The first step of the reaction sequence leading from glycine to serine (Scheme 11.9 in Chapter 11) provides a second example of attack on an aldehydic carbon, this time in the activated form of an imminium derivative. The key step in the context of the present discussion is that shown in Scheme 12.8. In view of what was said in the last chapter about the possible catalytic effect of the tetrahydrofolate coenzyme in this process it should be noted that the equivalent reaction with acetaldehyde can take place without the assistance of the second coenzyme.

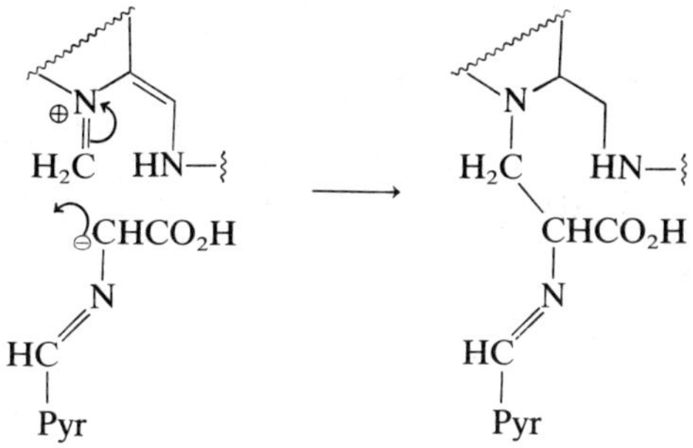

SCHEME 12.8

Biosynthesis of δ-aminolaevulinic acid. δ-Aminolaevulinic acid is an intermediate in porphyrin biosynthesis. It is generated as shown in Scheme 12.9 by condensation of succinyl CoA (derived from the citric acid cycle) with the carbanion derived from glycine. Once again the mechanism involves nucleophilic attack at carbon, leading in this case to displacement of a thiol residue. In the intermediate [100] the new (ketonic) carbonyl group is generated β to the carboxylic acid function of the amino acid residue and consequently the decarboxylation to produce the final product [101] is facilitated in the usual way.

Reactions involving β-elimination

The reactions which come under this heading are necessarily limited to those amino acids which possess a potential leaving group in the β-position. In general, after formation of the usual carbanion derivative,

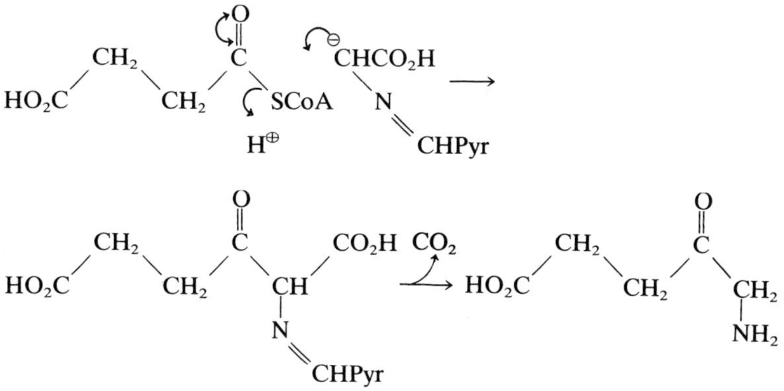

[100]　　　　　　　　　　　　[101]

SCHEME 12.9

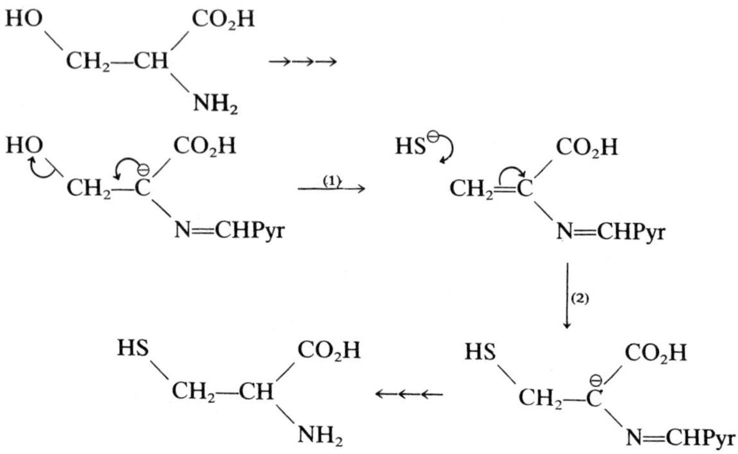

HO—CH$_2$—CH(CO$_2$H)(NH$_2$) →→→

HO—CH$_2$—C(CO$_2$H)(N=CHPyr)   —(1)→   HS$^{\ominus}$ CH$_2$=C(CO$_2$H)(N=CHPyr)

$\downarrow$ (2)

HS—CH$_2$—CH(CO$_2$H)(NH$_2$)   ←←←   HS—CH$_2$—C$^{\ominus}$(CO$_2$H)(N=CHPyr)

SCHEME 12.10

the leaving group is eliminated to give an α,β-unsaturated acid as in step (1) of Scheme 12.10.

This intermediate can then react by two entirely different mechanisms. The first involves addition of a nucleophile to regenerate a carbanion on the α-carbon. An important example of this type of reaction is shown in the continuation of Scheme 12.10; here the nucleophile is the sulphydryl anion and the ultimate product cysteine. Taking the scheme as a whole, the coenzyme can be considered as providing a neat way of avoiding the kinetic barrier to direct displacement of the hydroxyl group by a sulphydryl (for example in an S_N2 reaction).

Another reaction which follows this pattern is the generation of tryptophan [102] from serine. In this case the nucleophile is C-3 of indole. The relevant steps, corresponding to those from step (2) onwards in Scheme 12.10, are shown in Scheme 12.11.

The second type of transformation which hinges on a β-elimination mechanism is shown in Scheme 12.12. Here the coenzyme is cleaved from the intermediate α,β-unsaturated acid (step 1) to give an enamine which can protonate on the β-carbon (step 2) leading eventually by standard chemical steps to an α-keto acid. In its overall result this transformation corresponds to an internal redox reaction in which an oxidation takes place at the α-carbon at the expense of a reduction at the β-carbon.

Reactions in which pyridoxal is converted to pyridoxamine

In all the reactions discussed so far the coenzyme has played an essentially passive role, i.e. that of acting as an electron sink, and all the

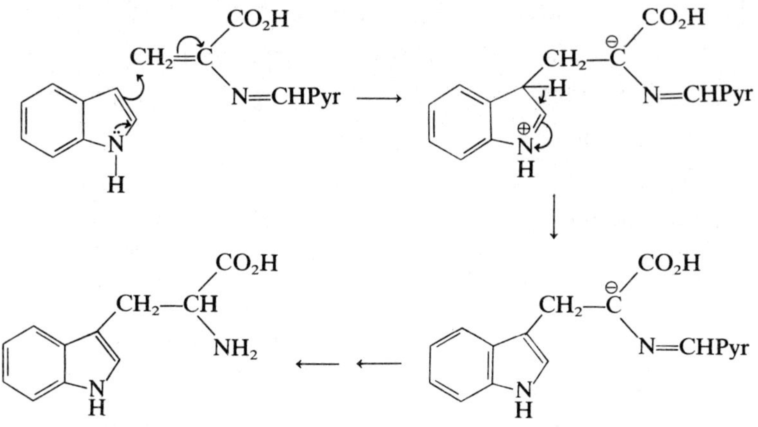

SCHEME 12.11

important electronic shifts could be considered to take place in the substrate residue. However, in the reactions to be discussed in this section the coenzyme is converted to a pyridoxamine [93] derivative. This structural change is brought about by protonation of the usual carbanion intermediate on the 'aldehyde carbon' of the coenzyme residue as shown in Scheme 12.13. As a result the α-carbon of the amino acid residue is oxidized to the ketone level and the intermediate [103] is the pyridoxamine derivative of an α-keto acid. Two fundamentally different amino acid transformations depend on this strategy, i.e. γ-elimination and α-oxidation, and they will be discussed in turn below.

γ-Elimination: homocysteine to α-ketobutyric acid. Overall this reaction can be viewed as an internal redox reaction in which the α-position of an amino acid is oxidized at the expense of the γ-position. Indeed this is how the reaction was listed earlier (reaction 6 in Scheme 12.1).

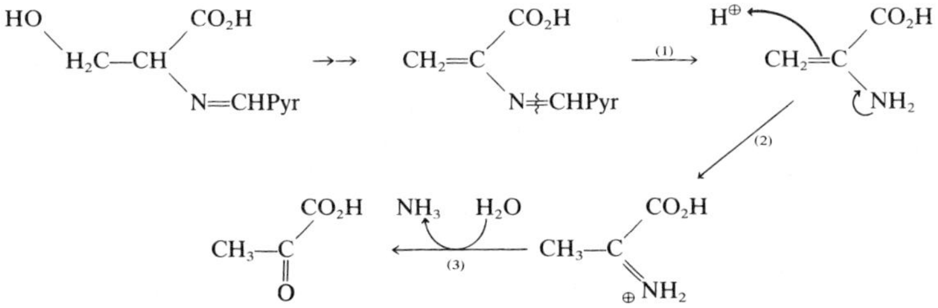

SCHEME 12.12

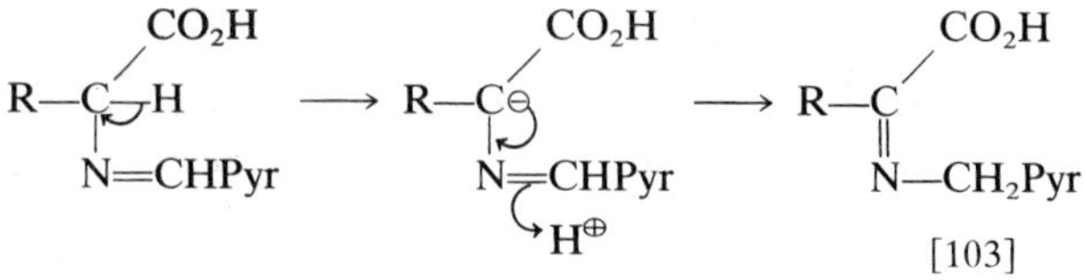

$$\text{R--}\underset{\underset{\text{N}=\text{CHPyr}}{|}}{\overset{\nearrow\text{CO}_2\text{H}}{\text{C}\diagdown\text{H}}} \longrightarrow \text{R--}\underset{\underset{\overset{\text{N}=\text{CHPyr}}{\diagdown\text{H}^{\oplus}}}{|}}{\overset{\nearrow\text{CO}_2\text{H}}{\text{C}\ominus}} \longrightarrow \text{R--}\underset{\text{N--CH}_2\text{Pyr}}{\overset{\nearrow\text{CO}_2\text{H}}{\text{C}}}$$

[103]

SCHEME 12.13

The mechanism proposed in Scheme 12.14 begins in steps (1) and (2) with the formation of the pyridoxamine derivative. Conversion of the imine group in the latter to an enamine (step 3) triggers the elimination of the thiol residue from the γ-position (step 4). In step (5) a 1,5-shift of a proton leads to regeneration of a pyridoxal derivative. The coenzyme is now cleaved from the substrate residue in the usual way (step 6) to give an enamine. The latter hydrolyses by standard reactions to the final product (cf. steps 1, 2 and 3 of Scheme 12.12). Hence we have now seen how the pyridoxal coenzyme can induce, in appropriately substituted amino acids, reaction at the α-position (e.g. in Scheme 12.5), the β-position (Scheme 12.10), and the γ-position (Scheme 12.14) of the carbon skeleton.

Interconversion of an amino acid with an α-keto acid. In this transformation, the second type that hinges on the formation of a pyridoxamine derivative, an amino acid is oxidized to an α-keto acid by an external agent. The oxidizing agent is a second α-keto acid, and, since the redox reaction is accompanied by amino group transfer, the product of its

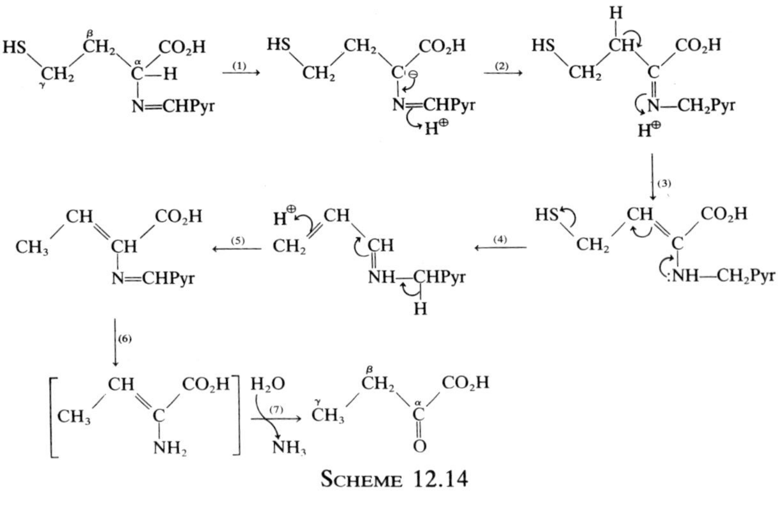

SCHEME 12.14

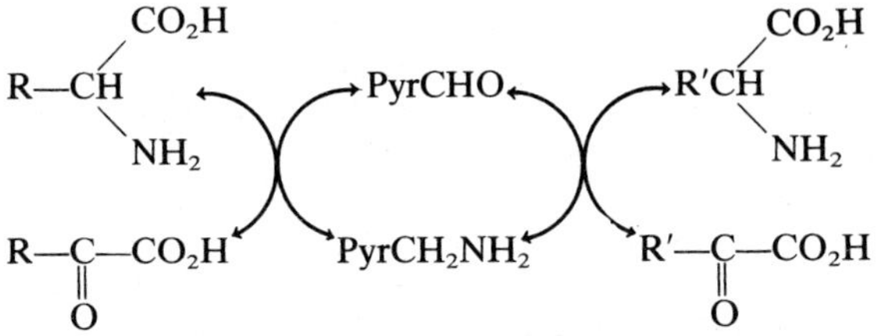

$$
\begin{array}{c}
\text{R—CH} \overset{\text{CO}_2\text{H}}{\underset{\text{NH}_2}{|}} \quad \rightleftharpoons \quad \text{PyrCHO} \quad \rightleftharpoons \quad \text{R'CH} \overset{\text{CO}_2\text{H}}{\underset{\text{NH}_2}{|}} \\
\\
\text{R—C—CO}_2\text{H} \quad\quad \text{PyrCH}_2\text{NH}_2 \quad\quad \text{R'—C—CO}_2\text{H} \\
\overset{\parallel}{\text{O}} \quad\quad\quad\quad\quad\quad\quad\quad\quad\quad \overset{\parallel}{\text{O}}
\end{array}
$$

SCHEME 12.15

reduction is the corresponding amino acid. Typically the process operates in a cycle as shown in Scheme 12.15. It is readily reversible and therefore provides a means of interconverting a given pair of amino acids with the corresponding keto acids. As we shall see this is a vital part of amino acid metabolism.

The coenzyme normally remains bound throughout the cycle to one enzyme where it reacts in succession with the two substrates. Hence, although it is shown for simplicity as a free aldehyde at the top of the cycle, at that stage it is probably bound to the enzyme in the usual way as an imine derivative of lysine.

The main stages of one half of the cycle, including the key prototropic shift (step 2), are presented in Scheme 12.16. The steps are of standard types whose mechanisms have been discussed adequately already. In the second half of the cycle the reactions of Scheme 12.16 merely go into reverse with the second keto acid. Note that in this cycle the coenzyme serves as a carrier of hydrogen and an amino group from one substrate to another, and so, in contrast with earlier examples, it functions as more than a catalyst to facilitate electronic shifts in the substrate.

Oxidative deamination of primary amines. This reaction, in which a primary amine is oxidized to an aldehyde (reaction 8 of Scheme 12.1), can be regarded as a variant of that discussed above, for again a $CHNH_2$

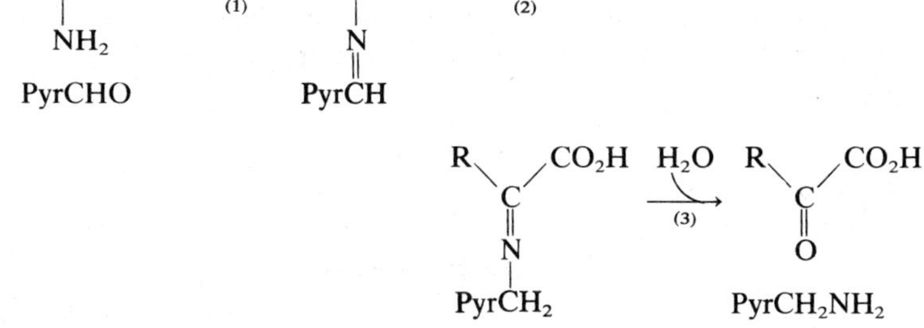

$$
\begin{array}{ccc}
\text{R} \diagdown \underset{\text{NH}_2}{\underset{|}{\overset{\diagup \text{CO}_2\text{H}}{\text{CH}}}} & \xrightarrow[\text{(1)}]{\text{H}_2\text{O}} & \text{R} \diagdown \underset{\text{PyrCH}}{\underset{\parallel}{\underset{\text{N}}{\overset{\diagup \text{CO}_2\text{H}}{\text{CH}}}}} \quad \xrightarrow{\text{(2)}} \\
\text{PyrCHO}
\end{array}
$$

$$
\begin{array}{ccc}
\text{R} \diagdown \underset{\text{PyrCH}_2}{\underset{|}{\underset{\text{N}}{\overset{\diagup \text{CO}_2\text{H}}{\underset{\parallel}{\text{C}}}}}} & \xrightarrow[\text{(3)}]{\text{H}_2\text{O}} & \text{R} \diagdown \underset{\text{PyrCH}_2\text{NH}_2}{\underset{\parallel}{\underset{\text{O}}{\overset{\diagup \text{CO}_2\text{H}}{\text{C}}}}}
\end{array}
$$

SCHEME 12.16

group in the substrate is converted to a carbonyl group. It probably follows the same general course as the reaction shown in Scheme 12.16 but with hydrogen in place of carboxyl. The subsequent stages are markedly different, however, for in this case the pyridoxamine is reoxidized to pyridoxal by molecular oxygen rather than by a keto acid. The mechanism of the reoxidation is not known. One interesting pointer, however, is the presence of copper in the enzymes in question, which may be the essential mediator in the reaction between molecular oxygen and the reduced coenzyme. In this connection it is interesting to recall from Chapter 6 that amino acids can also be oxidatively deaminated in a similar way at the expense of molecular oxygen but with the assistance of a flavoprotein rather than pyridoxal phosphate. It seems odd, in view of the dominant position of the latter coenzyme in amino acid metabolism, that it should be neglected in favour of the former one for this key reaction, but presumably this state of affairs is the consequence of no more than a chance development in the course of evolution.

The facility of these oxidative deamination reactions provides a tantalizing challenge to the organic chemist, for the transformation of a primary amino group to a carbonyl is a potentially useful synthetic transformation, and yet until recently there was no really reliable and convenient method for carrying it out *in vitro*. In essence what is required is a method of oxidizing a primary amine to an imine, because the subsequent deamination will normally take place spontaneously in aqueous solution. The scarcity of reliable methods for bringing about this transformation makes a striking contrast with the abundance of reagents which are available to bring about the equivalent redox reaction in the oxygen series, that is, the oxidation of a carbinol to a carbonyl group.

The desire to fill this gap has stimulated much research and since the discovery of the mechanism of action of pyridoxal phosphate in equivalent biological reactions there have been many attempts to develop a useful preparative method based on the same principle. The general strategy is shown in Scheme 12.17. The amine is condensed with an aldehyde to give an imine; this is then converted to the isomeric imine by a 1,3 shift of a proton via a carbanion intermediate, and finally the desired carbonyl compound is liberated by hydrolysis.

$$RCH_2NH_2 + R'CHO \xrightarrow{H_2O} RCH_2{-}N{=}CHR' \rightleftharpoons$$

$$RCH{=}N{-}CH_2{-}R' \xrightarrow{H_2O} RCHO + R'CH_2NH_2$$

SCHEME 12.17

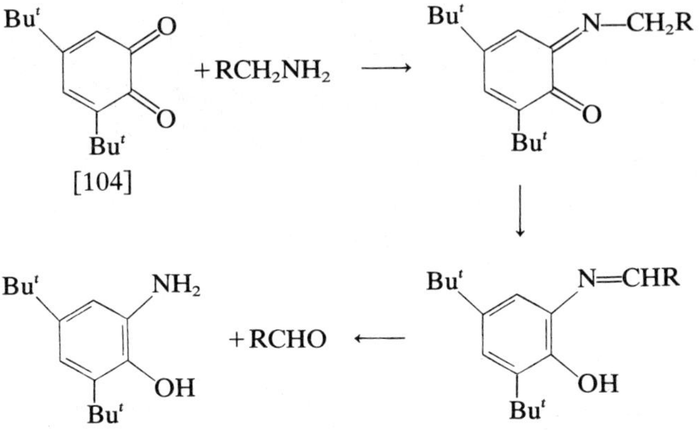

SCHEME 12.18

The approach is straightforward in principle but unfortunately it is difficult to achieve a useful preparative result in practice. Apart from various side-reactions (the nature of which depend on R and R') there is the problem of driving the interconversion of the imines in the desired direction. Several neat solutions to this problem have been devised and one of these is presented in Scheme 12.18 where the *o*-quinone [104] serves as the oxidizing agent. In the resulting imine the desired proton shift will go virtually to completion because it leads to aromatization of a quinonoid ring, and so there is a high overall conversion of the amine to the required carbonyl compound.

With this and similar reagents it is now possible to oxidize a primary amine under very mild conditions. Nevertheless we have probably not seen the final solution to this problem for, compared with the biological reaction, all the chemical methods reported so far suffer from a serious limitation: the oxidizing agent, which is expensive, is consumed in the process. Clearly it would be a major improvement to design a method where the oxidizing agent could be recycled *in situ*, as it is in the enzyme-mediated reaction, by oxidation with a readily available agent such as molecular oxygen. On that challenging note we conclude our survey of the chemical aspects of pyridoxal phosphate reactions.

Metabolic role of pyridoxal phosphate reactions

We shall now consider how the various reactions catalysed by pyridoxal phosphate are integrated into the overall plan of metabolism. The coenzyme mediates in two essentially different types of reaction. Firstly, there are reactions in which the carbon skeleton of an amino acid is assembled or degraded; secondly, there are reactions in which the

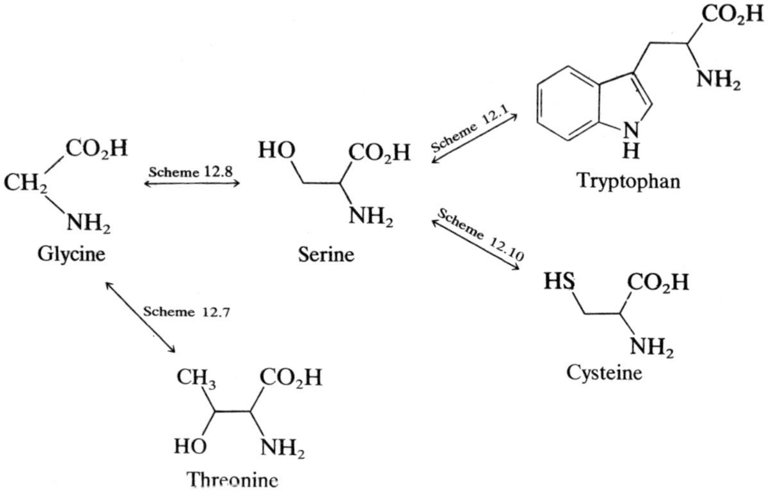

SCHEME 12.19

coenzyme assists in the introduction of an amino group to (or its removal from) a preformed carbon skeleton.

We have met several transformations which come into the first category and they are assembled in Scheme 12.19 in the form of a flowsheet which shows how glycine serves as a basic building block for a range of amino acids.

Turning to the second category, by far the most important reaction is the reductive amination of an α-keto acid. For example, the final step of phenylalanine biosynthesis involves reductive amination of a preformed skeleton in the form of phenylpyruvic acid (Scheme 12.20) with glutamic acid serving as the source of nitrogen. The list of amino acids which can be synthesized along these lines includes alanine (from pyruvic acid) and aspartic acid (from oxaloacetic acid). Transformations of this type are reversible and so they can readily serve as the first step of a catabolic sequence.

$$\mathrm{PhCH_2COCO_2H + HO_2CCH_2CH_2CH(NH_2)CO_2H \rightleftharpoons PhCH_2CH(NH_2)CO_2H + HO_2CCH_2CH_2COCO_2H}$$

SCHEME 12.20

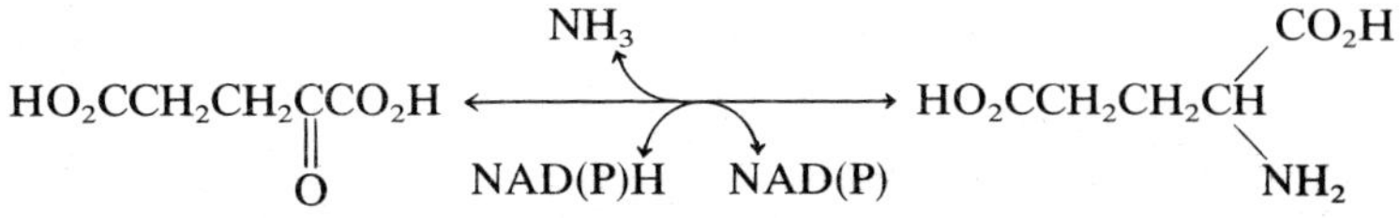

$$\text{HO}_2\text{CCH}_2\text{CH}_2\overset{\displaystyle \text{O}}{\underset{\displaystyle \text{O}}{\text{C}}}\text{CO}_2\text{H} \xleftarrow{\hspace{1cm}}\overset{\displaystyle \text{NH}_3}{\underset{\displaystyle \text{NAD(P)H} \quad \text{NAD(P)}}{\xrightarrow{\hspace{2cm}}}} \text{HO}_2\text{CCH}_2\text{CH}_2\overset{\displaystyle \text{CO}_2\text{H}}{\underset{\displaystyle \text{NH}_2}{\text{CH}}}$$

SCHEME 12.21

It must be emphasized however that reactions such as that shown in Scheme 12.20 do not provide a means for the *de novo* synthesis of amino acids, for all they achieve is a redistribution of the nitrogen already bound to carbon in the amino acid pool from one amino acid to another; what is needed in addition is a process by means of which 'free' nitrogen in the form of ammonia can be converted to 'bound' nitrogen in the pool of amino acids. Only a few reactions are known which can achieve this result. The most important is presented in Scheme 12.21 which shows how α-ketoglutarate can undergo reductive amination to form glutamic acid.

The keto acid is readily available as an intermediate of the citric acid cycle and consequently this reaction allows the pool of bound nitrogen to be increased or decreased according to the prevailing need. In this connection it is significant that both of the nicotinamide coenzymes can take part in the process. Presumably when there is need to increase the pool of bound nitrogen NADPH will be supplied so that amino acid synthesis will take place; when the call is for amino acid breakdown (as is the case, for example, in an animal on a protein-rich diet) the process is driven in the reverse direction by supplying NAD^+ instead. Hence we find once again the two nicotinamide enzymes exercising control over the direction of operation of a key metabolic reaction.

Taking Schemes 12.20 and 12.21 together it becomes clear that glutamic acid can be viewed as a carrier of nitrogen from the free pool of ammonia to that bound in the phenylalanine pool. It is significant that the enzymes which carry out the type of transformation shown in Scheme 12.20 normally accept glutamic acid as one of the two substrates and so this amino acid plays a wide-ranging role in the distribution of bound nitrogen through the amino acid pool.

Tracing metabolic relationships

As a concluding exercise it is instructive to examine briefly how some of the amino acid pathways interlock with the central pathways discussed in earlier chapters. Accordingly a rudimentary metabolic pathways map has been assembled in Scheme 12.22. All the reactions and pathways shown have been considered in detail at some stage of this book.

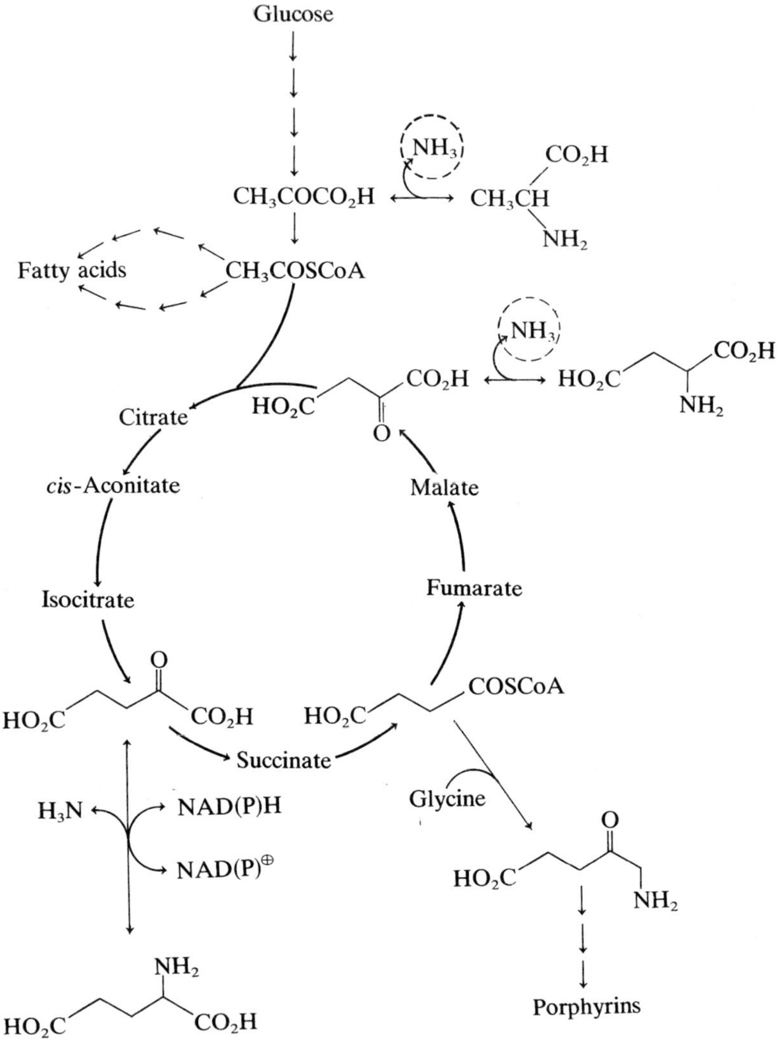

SCHEME 12.22

    The pathways of glycolysis and the citric acid cycle (shown in outline only) provide the core of the diagram and it is clear why they can justifiably be called the central pathways. Apart from their role in the provision of energy they can be seen to provide the raw material for a variety of biosyntheses and also to receive the end-products of several catabolic pathways.

Alanine is formed from pyruvic acid, and two citric acid cycle intermediates oxaloacetate and α-ketoglutarate are similarly used to produce amino acids, subject of course to replacement material being provided by a suitable anaplerotic pathway. In presenting these reactions a distinction is drawn between the one which uses free ammonia (bottom left) and those which use 'bound' nitrogen provided by glutamic acid (indicated for simplicity by NH_3 in a dotted circle). Also succinyl CoA is shown reacting with glycine as the first step of porphyrin biosynthesis.

Although the scheme presents no more than a small fraction of the metabolic pathways map it helps to illustrate the principles which underly its design and hopefully the reader will now feel sufficiently confident and interested to delve more deeply into this complex and fascinating subject.

Suggestions for further reading

Comprehensive Biochemistry Textbooks

LEHNINGER, A. L. (1970) *Biochemistry*, Worth, New York.

MAHLER, H. R. and CORDES, E. H. (1971) *Biological chemistry* (2nd edn.) HARPER and ROW, New York.

A Survey of the Metabolic Pathways.

NICOLSON, D. E., and DAGLEY, S. (1970) *Introduction to metabolic pathways*, Blackwell, Oxford.

Chemical Models for Enzyme Catalysis

JENCKS, W. P. (1969) *Catalysis in chemistry and enzymology*, McGraw-Hill, New York.

BRUICE, T. C. and BENKOVIC, S. J. (1966) *Bioorganic mechanisms*, Benjamin, New York.

The Catalytic Groups of Enzymes

GRAY, C. J. (1971) *Enzyme catalysed reactions*, Reinhold, London.

SMELLIE, R. M. S. (ed.) (1970) *Chemical reactivity and biological role of functional groups in enzymes*, Academic Press, London.

Index

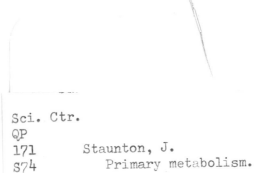